EATING FOR A's

EATING FOR A's

A month-by-month nutrition and lifestyle guide
to help raise smarter kids

Kindergarten to 6th grade

Kathleen M. Dunn, MPH, RD
Lorna A. Williams, MPH, RD

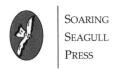

SOARING
SEAGULL
PRESS

Eating for A's
A month-by-month nutrition and lifestyle guide to help raise smarter kids

Published by
Soaring Seagull Press
PO Box 48, Santa Rosa CA 95402
www.EatingFor.com

Although every precaution has been taken in the preparation of this book, the authors and publisher assume no responsibility for errors or omissions. The authors and publisher expressly disclaim any responsibility for any liability, loss, injury or risk, personal or otherwise, which is incurred as a consequence, directly or indirectly, of the use and application of any of the contents of this book.

The information in this book is provided for educational purposes and general reference. It is not meant to be a substitute for medical advice or counseling. Consult a physician before making any changes to diet, exercise or other health habits as described in this book.

All trademarks and photographs are the property of their respective owners. Photograph on page 10 courtesy of Oakland Athletics; pages 18, 90, 218 and 288 by Cathy Yeulet / Bigstock.com; pages 36, 144, 176 and 232 by Lorna Williams / Soaring Seagull Press; page 52 by Andres Rodriguez / Bigstock.com; pages 80 and 298 by Thomas Perkins / Bigstock.com; page 106 by Wavebreak Media Ltd / Bigstock.com; page 126 by Christophe Rolland / Bigstock.com; page 166 by Eli Mordechai / Bigstock.com; page 192 by Valeriy Lebedev / Bigstock.com; page 264 by Mandy Godbehear / Bigstock.com; page 308 by Daniel Hurst / Bigstock.com; and back cover by Katharine Noble.

Cover Design | Andy Paolella (www.andypao.com)
Illustrations | Lorna Williams, Anika Williams

Library of Congress Control Number: 2012905221
ISBN: 978-0-9848540-0-4

Printed in the United States of America

Dedication

To my husband Chris for his unwavering belief in this project and to the memory of my parents who taught me that achieving life's goals requires the right blend of good nutrition, hard work and confidence—all nourished by a kind heart.

– Kathleen Dunn, MPH, RD

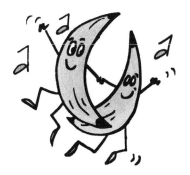

To my husband Brad for his endless support and encouragement, to my children Andrew and Anika who fill my world with joy and laughter and to my parents who lovingly taught me the secret of a life in balance—work hard (thanks, Dad), but remember to take time to dance (thanks, Mom).

– Lorna Williams, MPH, RD

Table of Contents

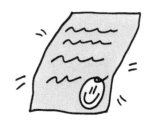

Part 1
Introduction

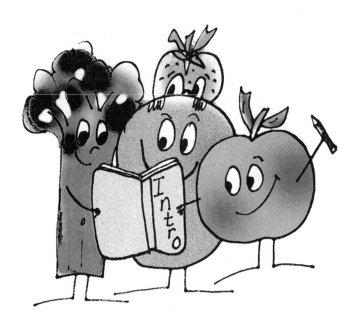

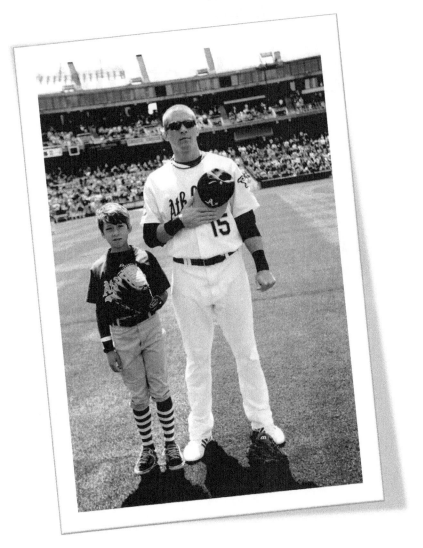

What we think, we become.
                        — Buddha

Chapter 1

Start Here

As registered dietitians, we've heard the collective battle cry from busy parents who want the best for their children: "Give us nutrition tips to help our kids excel in school. No information overload. No complex strategy to learn. Just the need-to-know basics that work with today's hectic lifestyle." If this sounds all too familiar, then this book is for you.

We listened and went to work distilling essential nutrition information into 12 goals that are sure to help your child build the healthy habits that an active mind and optimal learning demand.

Why 12 goals? For most parents of young children, it's second nature to juggle schedules around the months of a typical school year. September typically ushers in the excitement of a new school year, January marks the halfway point and June signals the beginning of long summer days. So, why not apply this same by-the-month mindset to shape healthy, brain-building habits for your kids? After all, behavioral scientists have found that it takes about 28 days to transform a new behavior into a regular habit. What's more, organizing each monthly goal around the activities of a typical school year lets you put them into practice in real life—your real life.

Work Smart, Not Hard

To get the most out of this book, we recommend that you concentrate on one chapter per month. This allows you plenty of time to put each chapter's goal into practice.

With each new chapter, you'll tackle a new goal, but you'll also continue practicing your new habits from previous chapters. With each month, you'll be one step closer to a solid foundation of 12 brain-boosting habits that will help your kids reach their full potential.

To coincide with the school year, start at the chapter that corresponds with the month during which you're reading. For example, if you start reading this book in September, begin with Chapter 2: September – Family Meals. If, however, you should open this book in the middle of the school year, say in January, we recommend that you start at Chapter 6: January – Pack a Power Lunch. In other words, there is no "best" time to start—unless it's now!

A word of caution: Don't be tempted to move ahead. Stay focused on tackling one chapter—and one goal—per month. If you're anxious to do more, explore the extra credit in each chapter. Remember, this is not a race against time; it's a day-to-day approach. The best way to win is with a slow and steady pace.

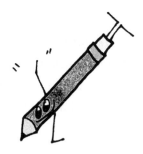

Tips from Parents

As you read, you'll notice each chapter includes "Parent Pearls." These are creative solutions we've learned from parents like you who are eager to encourage better food choices for the entire family, but especially for their young children.

Tips from Experts

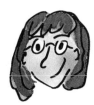

Each chapter also includes information on the latest scientific evidence from experts in the field of nutrition as it relates to each chapter's topic. You'll find these tidbits highlighted in the "Did You Know?" boxes throughout the book.

Setting Goals like a Pro

The best way to establish healthy habits is to set goals. Goals help us achieve what we want in life; they reflect our purpose and have a wide impact on our lives. Goals give our lives meaning. They are the stepping stones toward our dreams.

But, all too often, people set lofty goals that all but defy the basic laws of physiology and are sadly doomed to fail. "We're going to add five more servings of fruit to our daily menu." "We're going to double our fiber intake starting tomorrow." "We're going to eliminate all sugar starting tomorrow." As soon as we hear these grand proclamations from parents who are eager to improve their family's nutrition and lifestyle habits, we have a pretty good idea of the disappointment that lies ahead.

A better approach is to set reasonable goals that you're likely to achieve. Talk with your child and get their input. Encourage them to get a little out of their comfort zone. After all, it's only when we stretch the canvas of life that we can really reach our full potential.

Here's how you can set goals like the pros do. Every effective goal includes five key elements. They must be **S**pecific, **M**easurable, **A**ttainable, **R**ealistic and **T**imed. Behavior experts often refer to this type of goal by its acronym, a SMART goal. Read on for a quick primer on how to make sure your goals are SMART goals.

5 Elements of a SMART Goal

1 **A SMART goal is specific.** Let's say your child is on the chubby side, and the excess weight is a concern. For overweight kids, who are otherwise healthy, it's generally recommended to allow them to "grow" into their weight rather than put them on a weight loss diet, so a specific weight loss goal is generally not recommended. Rather, encourage your child to focus on the specific behaviors involved in achieving a healthy body weight and set goals related to those behaviors. For example, "I will replace my daily snack of potato chips with

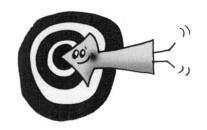

popcorn or a piece of fruit" or "I will put my fork down between bites."

2 **A SMART goal is measurable.** After all, how else can you evaluate your child's success unless you have something to measure? Here's a measurable goal to increase physical activity: "I'm going to walk three times for 30 minutes this week. Next week, I'll add a 5-minute stretch after each session." There's no doubt about whether or not you meet this goal because it's measurable.

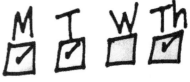

3 **A SMART goal is attainable.** To be sure, you must be able to achieve a goal using the resources available to you right now. For example, a goal aimed at serving your kids a wide variety of fresh fruits for after-school snacks may be difficult or even unattainable during those months when the selection is limited. But, a minor tweak that broadens your goal to include frozen fruits would make it more attainable throughout the year.

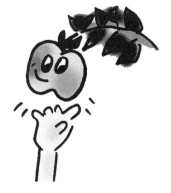

4 **A SMART goal is realistic.** With every goal you set, you should be willing to put in the effort needed to get out of your comfort zone, but don't overdo it. Goals that are too difficult are not only unrealistic, they can be downright frustrating. On the other hand, goals that are too easy typically lead to boredom. Realistic goals have just the right amount of challenge that fuels an "I can do this" attitude.

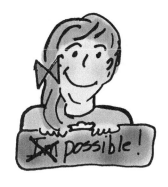

5 **A SMART goal is time sensitive.** Setting the deadline when you expect to achieve a goal is essential for success. Without establishing the time frame in which you expect to accomplish your goal—a meal, a day, a week—your goal is only a dream, and you're likely to travel down the "I'll do it tomorrow" road to failure. Of course, a deadline is also the perfect opportunity to evaluate your progress.

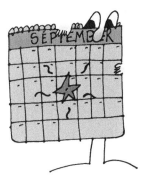

Go for the Goal!

To make it easier for you and your family, we have included suggested SMART goals for each month at the end of each chapter. These 12 goals represent a solid foundation for optimal physical and mental health. Meet these goals and your child's active mind and body will be nourished with the high-octane fuel that only sound nutrition can deliver. Inspired to do even more? You'll find "Extra Credit" goals in each chapter to create even more healthy habits.

Before you start, we encourage you to give some serious thought about what you and your child really want to accomplish this year. The more thought you put into setting SMART goals, the better you'll help your child succeed. And, for easier goal tracking, you'll find plenty of **My Smart Tracker** forms in Chapter 14: Go for the Goal! ready and waiting for you to track your success. Let's get started!

Part 2
Fall Days

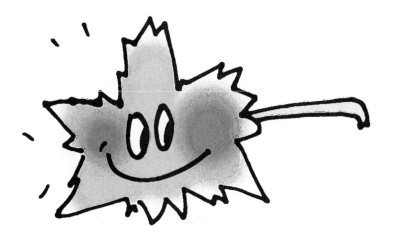

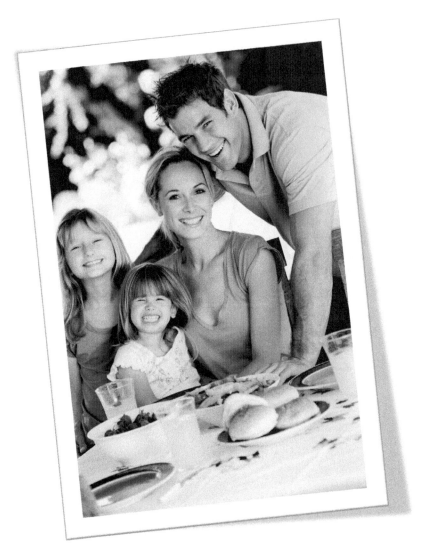

Eating is not merely a material pleasure. Eating well gives a spectacular joy to life and contributes immensely to goodwill and happy companionship. It is of great importance to the morale.
— *Elsa Schiaparelli*

Chapter 2

September – Family Meals

For most children, September kicks off a new school year, and the new routine is a perfect time to focus on healthy—and happy—family meals. In fact, of all the healthy behaviors worth making a regular habit, few are more important for boosting your little one's brainpower than sitting down together to enjoy a healthy meal and engaging conversation.

Child development experts agree: Make the family meal a regular habit, and children are more likely to grow up happier, healthier and well adjusted. They're also more likely to eat fruits, vegetables and other nutrient-rich foods and less likely to drink sugary soft drinks and other empty-calorie foods.

Trouble is, for many parents of young children, September also brings daily schedules that border on superhuman. Alarm clocks are set earlier for the new morning routine. Shuttling the kids to and from school, sports activities, music, dance and art lessons becomes a full-time job. And, motivating their active minds to start—and finish—homework becomes a nightly ritual. That's on top of an already hectic work day. With today's jam-packed schedules, it's easy to see how the family meal can fall by the wayside.

The good news is, you can reclaim your family meals. It's easier than you may think and well worth the effort. After all, shaping the healthy habit of regular family meals is not only linked to better academic performance, but it also helps keep your kids out of trouble.

As younger kids become pre-teens and teenagers, sitting down to frequent family dinners becomes a protective factor that helps curtail a wide variety of high-risk behaviors, according to a study published in the *Journal of Adolescent Health*. In this study, University of Minnesota researchers surveyed over 99,000 sixth to 12th graders in 200 cities across the United States and found a consistent link between frequent family dinners and a reduced risk of all high-risk behaviors measured—all of them—including substance abuse, sexual promiscuity, depression, suicide, antisocial behaviors, violence, school problems and eating disorders.

Family meals are also linked to stronger family bonds and better diet quality. What's more, families that eat regular family meals tend to maintain leaner, healthier body weights. Ready to get started? Read on for the need-to-know essentials to make brain-boosting family meals part of your daily routine.

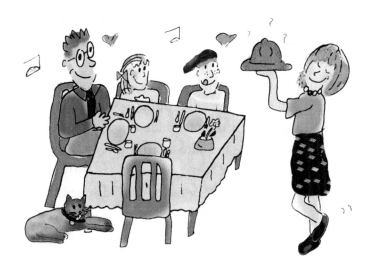

10 Easy Steps for Great Family Meals

1 **Aim for five family meals each week.** With today's hectic, overscheduled lifestyles, the real challenge for most families is to make the family meal the rule rather than the exception. Researchers recommend sitting down to an enjoyable family meal at least five times a week. That's the number of occurrences found to have the most positive impact on a child's health and well-being. Start tracking how many times your family eats together. If it's less than five times each week, focus on adding one meal per week until you achieve this goal. If your family sits down to at least five family meals each week, congratulate yourself. You're on track!

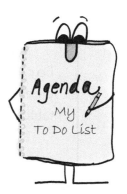

2 **Plan to eat together.** The most common barrier to family meals is busy or conflicting schedules, especially when parents have work schedules that allow little flexibility and kids have activities with strict attendance requirements. The solution is to treat family meals like any other important appointment. Find your calendar now, and schedule your family meals—remember, aim for at least five per week—to be sure you keep this important commitment.

3 **Choose solutions that fit your schedule.** If you can't avoid scheduling sports practice, dance classes or other activities for the kids during your typical dinner hour, plan a simple tailgate or bleacher dinner before practice. Remember, you don't need to cook from scratch, dine at a fancy table or eat from the good china. You just need to eat a healthy meal and enjoy each other's company. If dinner is a challenge due to work schedules, consider scheduling regular family breakfasts to achieve your goal of at least five family meals each week. A Sunday morning family breakfast is an ideal, relaxing option. Get the kids involved. You may be surprised at their creative solutions.

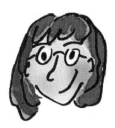

Did You Know?

The fourth Monday in September is National Family Day. This national initiative was developed to remind parents that the one thing kids really want at the dinner table is you.

For more information and inspiration about what you can do to celebrate, visit www.casafamilyday.org.

4 **Avoid using food as bribes or rewards.** This rule is especially true for younger children. "Eat your peas, and you can have ice cream," may earn you a few bites from your 5-year-old, but it's unlikely to encourage your child to ask for peas again. This type of bribe may seem harmless, but it actually teaches kids to associate certain foods with rewards. Trouble is, these "reward" foods are typically high in fat and sugar and low in brain-building nutrients.

5 **Avoid rushing.** Allow plenty of time to enjoy a family meal that's relaxing; aim for at least 30 minutes. After all, rushing reinforces two not-so-good habits—eating too fast and eating too much—which can lead to upset tummies after the meal and excess weight gain over the long run.

6 **Have patience with manners.** Remind your kids to mind their manners, but avoid being too rigid. Use our 1:2 Rule: For every manner in need of reminding—"Elbows off the table," "Sit up straight," "Don't slurp," "Use your fork," "Don't talk with a full mouth"—praise your kids for two they did without reminding.

7 **Create a welcoming experience.** The family meal is more than just about serving healthy foods; it's also about creating an enjoyable, relaxed, welcoming experience. No need to break the bank. Convenient, inexpensive solutions are everywhere from candles or flowers for the table to colorful paper plates or placemats to cheerful napkins. Your special touch is sure to make family meals more welcoming. If kids look forward to a family meal, they're more likely to be open to eating their favorite healthy foods and more likely to try new ones.

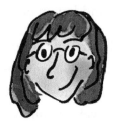

Did You Know?

Sitting down to frequent family meals gives your kids an edge in so many ways. Here are just a few of the advantages of regular family meals:

- Stronger family ties
- More nutritious diet
- Healthier body weight
- Less substance abuse and other high-risk behaviors

Researchers recommend you aim for at least five family meals each week. Don't forget, all meals count.

8 **Unplug for 30 minutes.** Turn the TV off, banish electronic games during the meal, let voicemail pick up phone calls and focus on conversation. With the typical meal lasting about 30 minutes, unplugging during mealtime is doable even for the most sophisticated techies among us— kids and adults alike.

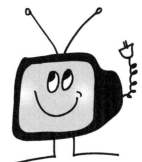

9 **Talk it up.** Engage everyone in conversation. Talking, not the food, should be the focus. Keep the conversation positive, encouraging and upbeat. Focus on positive topics such as "What did you do today to make it a good day?" Avoid arguments and save potentially stressful subjects for a non-meal time.

10 **Banish the clean plate club.** If your child refuses to eat broccoli, don't pressure and don't make a big deal about it. Be sure to offer it again at another meal, perhaps at several meals, but avoid pressure. Remember, your goal is to offer nutritious foods so your kids have plenty from which to choose.

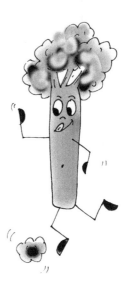

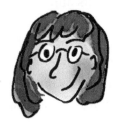

Did You Know?

You can teach your kids a smarter way to use their homework time. Here's how: Simply decide on the amount of time to spend on each subject before your child starts. For example, if your daughter has 45 minutes to tackle her homework, she could decide to spend 20 minutes on algebra, 15 minutes on language and 10 minutes to review for a spelling test.

Not only do kids learn a valuable lesson in budgeting their time, but they'll use that time more efficiently.

What's for Dinner?

For most families, dinner is the best time for family meals. Don't worry, it doesn't have to be complicated or time consuming. It doesn't even have to be home cooked. Simple, delicious meals planned together are the best.

Get the family involved by allowing each person to choose a favorite menu for at least one meal each week. Even young children have a favorite main dish, vegetable and fruit to plan a meal around. Keep things interesting by occasionally adding a new food for the family to try. You never know when you'll stumble on a new favorite.

When you plan and schedule family meals, you'll also reap the benefits that anticipation provides. When kids know when and what to expect for the meal, they feel more secure, avoid grazing on junk food before the meal and come to the table hungry, but not starving, to better enjoy the nutritious foods you serve.

Don't Forget Breakfast

As mentioned, breakfast can be another opportunity for a family meal. What's more, eating a healthy breakfast gets your child's day started off on the right foot and boosts learning. Shape this healthy behavior when your kids are young, and they'll be more likely to make it a daily habit as they age.

Parent Pearl

Set an appreciation plate. As a family, we sometimes set a special place setting at the dinner table to spotlight one family member. During the meal, each person shares what they appreciate about the mealtime star. Everyone benefits from the feel-good nature of positive sharing.

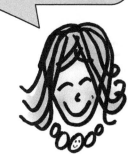

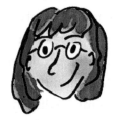

Did You Know?

Multivitamins are easier on the stomach and better absorbed when taken with food. So, encourage your child to take a multi with a meal—every day.

By giving your child a complete multivitamin every day, you help guard against food jags, finicky eating and half-eaten lunches. It's a type of dietary insurance that helps ensure your child is getting the nutrients needed to stay focused and sharp all day long.

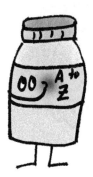

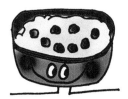

For those mornings when your routine is already jam-packed, a ready-in-minutes breakfast is ideal to fuel hungry minds with essential nutrients for learning. A hot bowl of oatmeal with fruit and nuts, whole wheat toast topped with peanut butter and applesauce or whole grain toaster waffles with fresh fruit and a glass of milk are just a few no-fuss solutions to start the day right.

Meal Time is Multi Time

Be sure to fill the nutrient gap between what your child is eating and what their growing body and active brain actually need with a daily multivitamin.

High-quality multivitamins designed to please even the most finicky kids are readily available from squishy gummies to chewable cartoon characters to flavored liquids and sour tarts. Choose your favorite, but make sure it's a complete multivitamin developed just for kids to ensure the proper amount of essential nutrients, including this important mineral. Iron is the most common nutrient deficiency among children, yet it's critical for learning. So, be sure to choose a multi that provides at least 100 percent of the Daily Value of iron.

Once you've found a favorite, shape a regular habit so your child remembers to take a multi every day. We recommend taking a daily multi at breakfast. It's an easy routine to get into, it fuels the day with added nutrition, and you don't have to think about it the rest of the day!

Parent Pearl

Whip up a healthy breakfast. My kids gobble up my fast-scrambled eggs. I beat two eggs together with ¼ cup milk in a micro-wavable dish and microwave for about 2 minutes. It rises like a soufflé. Fluff with a fork and sprinkle with low-fat cheese. I serve with whole wheat toast with jam and low-fat milk, and the kids are ready to start their day.

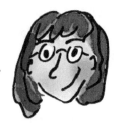

Did You Know?

Looking for a quick and brainy tailgate meal? Here are five no-fuss ideas to try:

1. Thermos of soup accompanied with a hearty whole grain roll.
2. Sandwich fixings packed in a pita pocket.
3. Ready-made rotisserie chicken with a pre-packed salad.
4. An upgraded peanut butter and jelly sandwich. Add sliced banana, cut into finger-sized portions and serve with sliced oranges, grapes, strawberries or other small fruits.
5. Whole grain crackers with hummus or sliced cheese and luncheon meats accompanied by a fruit salad.

TV Advertising & Brain Drain

It's no surprise that brain-building foods typically fail to top the list of foods and beverages advertised to children on television. In fact, it's just the opposite. The Institute of Medicine's Food and Nutrition Board recently confirmed that food advertising to young children is geared to entice kids with high-fat, sugary foods and beverages with little or no nutritional value, according to their report, *Food Marketing to Children and Youth: Threat or Opportunity?*

Adding insult to injury is the growing body of research that confirms the power that television advertising has over young children, aged 2 to 11 years. Not only are kids likely to break their own piggy banks to buy the latest advertised treat, but they'll want you to empty your wallet to buy it for them. Researchers call this "influencing purchases and requests to buy." Parents know it as that all too familiar—and entirely too persistent— must-have-it nagging. This advertising power is especially troublesome for children 8 years and younger, who typically have difficulty understanding the persuasive intent of marketing messages.

To be sure, an occasional treat won't harm your child's growing brain, but the daily nagging can certainly chip away at your resolve to keep the amount of junk food in your child's diet to a minimum. The good news is research suggests that all this advertising only moderately affects a young child's beliefs about foods and beverages and their typical dietary intake. For the most part, the influence of

> **Parent Pearl**
>
> **Routine can rock.** Have your child put any special school projects and all homework in their backpack the night before and place it by the door. This simple routine helps prevent the forgetfulness that can occur during the morning dash out the door!

television advertising on young children is limited to short-term consumption. So, your challenge is to keep the whining at bay, while instilling healthy habits and food choices.

Simple Ways to Fight TV Advertising

1 **Be a good role model.** When it comes to shaping healthy habits in your kids, your actions speak volumes.

2 **Limit TV time.** This is especially true for commercial programming. The Stanford School of Medicine recommends no more than two hours per day, according to a 2007 report.

3 **Choose programming on non-commercial stations whenever possible.** This will help reduce exposure to ads for high-fat, sugary foods.

4 **Discuss marketing techniques with your kids.** This will help your children understand the persuasive intent of ads.

Parent Pearl

Schedule routine eye exams. Our pediatrician always mentions how important good eyesight is for optimal learning. So, I make sure I schedule a complete eye exam for each of my kids as part of our annual back-to-school preparations.

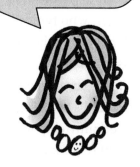

10 Quick & Brainy After-School Snacks

1. Fresh fruit (in season)
2. Macaroni & cheese
3. Popcorn
4. Pretzels
5. Pumpkin bread
6. Quesadilla (with whole wheat tortilla)
7. Fruit smoothie
8. Soybeans
9. String cheese
10. Walnuts and raisins

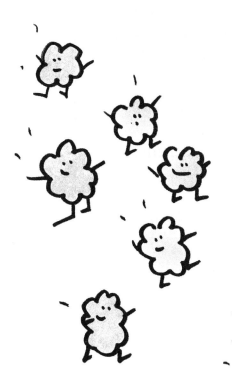

Parent Pearl

At breakfast, we use the cereal box to inspire a few brainteasers. How many adjectives start with the letter "S"? How much calcium is in one serving? What do you think inspired the name of the cereal? It's a great way to foster my child's reading and critical thinking skills.

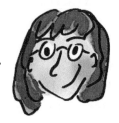

Did You Know?

Talking about the day's activities tops the list of benefits of family meals for most parents of school-aged kids, according to research published in the *Journal of the American Dietetic Association*. Researchers at the University of Minnesota surveyed over 100 parents of children, aged 8 to 10 years, to find out just what inspires them to make time for family meals. Here's the breakdown of the top reasons:

- Enjoying conversation and talking about the day
- Eating together, relaxing and laughing
- Enjoying good home-cooked food and nutritious, balanced meals
- Time to reconnect with the family
- Structured time together and time to plan other activities

This Month's Smart Goal

I will add one family meal each week to reach at least five per week. *

At least five is the goal, but for this goal and all others, make sure to set them for where you and your family are. Make sure your goals are not too hard, but not too easy either.

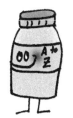

This Month's Extra Credit

I will give my child a children's multivitamin with 18 milligrams of iron every day, preferably at breakfast.

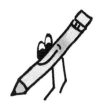

To monitor your daily progress toward your goals, use the **My Smart Tracker** forms in Chapter 14: Go for the Goal!

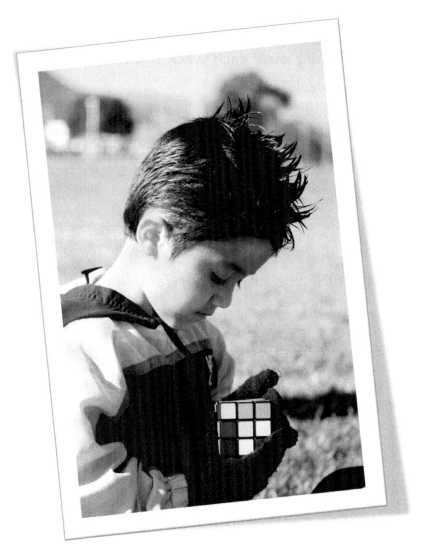

The brain is like a muscle. When it is in use,
we feel very good. Understanding is joyous.
— Carl Sagan

Chapter 3

October – Feed a Growing Brain

Of all the advantages you can give your child to help them excel, nourishing their brain is sure to rank among the most important. After all, when the brain is well-nourished, focused attention, eager learning and excellent grades are sure to follow. In this chapter, you'll learn what to look for when choosing the best brain foods for your rising star.

Foods that Activate Nerve Cells

Nerve cells—or neurons—communicate using a variety of chemical messengers called neurotransmitters. The signal starts when one neuron sends out a neurotransmitter to a neighboring neuron to spark it into action. The neighboring neuron does the same to its neighbor and so on. The signaling continues over a vast neural network that would rival the most complex metropolitan freeway system.

To make these important neurotransmitters, the body needs a steady supply of foods that contain protein. Why? Protein contains nitrogen-based compounds called amino acids, including the so-called essential amino acids that must be provided in the diet because the body is unable to synthesize them. Many amino acids, including some of the essential ones, serve as the building blocks for the body's production of neurotransmitters that are critical for learning and other brain functions.

How much protein does your child need for optimal learning? Aim for at least 19 grams of protein per day for younger kids, aged 4 to 8 years, and at least 34 grams per day for children aged 9 to 13 years.

The good news is many protein-rich foods are also kid-friendly foods, making it even easier to prepare meals and snacks. Read on for our top choices for brain-boosting protein foods.

Parent Pearl

Homework is a breeze in our house with a few simple rules. First, I encourage the kids to tackle the tough stuff when their confidence is high. Otherwise, they can breeze through easier assignments first. We also have a "stick-with-it" rule: The shortest amount of time to spend on a tough subject before switching gears.

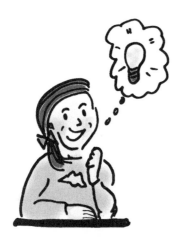

Protein-Rich Brain Foods

1 **Milk.** Each 1-cup serving provides **about 8 grams** of brain-boosting protein. Of course, white dairy milk is the kid-friendly staple, but don't forget the flavored varieties to entice finicky kids to drink up. Low-fat varieties are best for most healthy school-aged children. Fill the fridge with low-fat or fat-free milk products, especially if your kids tend to be on the heavier side. Non-dairy milk beverages such as soy milk or almond milk are also available and provide **about 6 to 8 grams** of protein per serving.

2 **Yogurt.** Each 6-ounce serving provides **about 8 grams** of protein. Like milk, low-fat varieties are available. And, with the seemingly endless variety of fruit and other flavors, you're sure to find a few that will make your little genius smile.

3 **Cheese.** Each 1-ounce serving provides **about 7 grams**, so you can't beat cheese for a protein boost. The next time you serve up a warm bowl of macaroni and cheese, a grilled cheese sandwich or other cheesy favorite, remember the brain-boosting benefits of cheese.

4 **Lean Meat, Fish and Poultry.** From lean hamburgers to fish fillets to grilled chicken, these protein-rich foods boast **about 7 grams** of protein per ounce. Aim for healthy portions—up to 2 ounces per serving, which is about the size of a ping pong ball.

> ### Parent Pearl
>
> **My on-the-go kids love yogurt.** So, I stock up on brands packaged for convenience such as low-fat yogurt in a tube. With no spoon required, it's a great choice for my nonstop kids.

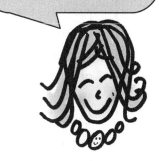

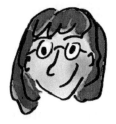

Did You Know?

You've probably heard the adage, "Breakfast is the most important meal of the day." We couldn't agree more. The word breakfast, literally means breaking the fast. After many hours without nourishment, breakfast provides important nutrients that fuel physical activity and mental performance during the morning hours. With food in the tummy, a child can focus on learning instead of on a rumbling stomach and what's on the lunch menu.

In a recent review of over 45 studies, researchers at the University of Florida found that kids who regularly eat breakfast may have the following advantages over their non-breakfast eating counterparts:

- Better brain power related to memory
- Better test grades
- Better school attendance
- Better overall diet
- Better health and sense of well-being
- Healthier body weight

Regularly eating breakfast makes sense—both for the brain and body. And, when it comes to breakfast, best bets are to choose a variety of foods, especially nutrient-rich whole grains, fruits and protein-rich foods. Bon appetite!

5 **Dried Beans, Peas and Lentils.** Kidney, navy, garbanzo and other dried beans as well as split green peas and hearty lentils are inexpensive nutrient wonders that pack **about 7 to 9 grams** of protein for each one-half cup serving. A warm bowl of chili, baked beans or other hearty bean dish is perfect for brisk October days.

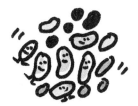

6 **Eggs.** Each egg provides **about 7 grams** of protein making it an ideal protein choice. Serve them scrambled with ketchup, poached over fiber-rich, whole-wheat toast, in a cheese omelet or hard-boiled for the lunch box. Healthy kids can enjoy eggs several times a week; however, children with high blood cholesterol may benefit from replacing whole eggs with egg whites, which are nearly all protein.

7 **Peanut Butter.** Peanut butter provides **about 4 grams** of protein per 1-tablespoon serving. It's a rare kid who doesn't love a delicious PB&J, a peanut butter filled celery boat or the occasional peanut butter cookie. For kids who just don't like peanut butter, many other "protein butter" options— almond, cashew, soy and more—are available that provide **about 3 to 4 grams** of protein per 1-tablespoon serving.

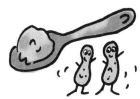

8 **Nuts and Seeds.** Almonds, cashews, peanuts, walnuts and other nuts provide between **4 to 7 grams** of protein per 1-ounce serving, or about 10 to 20 nuts, depending on the variety. Nuts are high in fat, so be sure to keep the serving size in check. Consider buying them in single-serving packages, which are perfect for on-the-go activities, lunch boxes and snacks.

9 **Whole Grains.** While not the protein powerhouse of other food groups, whole grain foods—brown rice, whole grain pasta, whole wheat bread and others—are still good sources with **about 3 grams** of protein per one-half cup or 1-ounce serving.

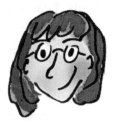

Did You Know?

Your child needs to consume choline every day for optimal brain health. How much? Young kids, aged 4 to 8 years, need at least 250 milligrams every day. Older kids, aged 9 to 13 years, need at least 375 milligrams every day. The good news is it's found in lots of kid favorites!

Food (Serving Size)	Choline (milligrams)
Egg (1 each)	100 mg
Cabbage, red, chopped (½ cup)	88 mg
Fish filet (3 ounces)	75 mg
Chicken breast (3 ounces)	72 mg
Hamburger (3 ounces)	71 mg
Soymilk (1 cup)	58 mg
Milk, 1% low-fat (1 cup)	43 mg
Soybeans, cooked (½ cup)	41 mg
Cauliflower, cooked (½ cup)	24 mg
Peanut butter (2 tablespoons)	20 mg
Peanuts (1 ounce)	15 mg
Wheat germ (1 tablespoon)	13 mg
Oatmeal, cooked (½ cup)	8 mg

Source: USDA Nutrient Database.

Foods that Shape Up Brain Cells

One of the hallmarks of a healthy cell is a pliable, flexible membrane ready and able to drink in the nutrients critical for peak performance and jettison toxins and metabolic byproducts that may cause harm. Your child's brain cells are no exception and will thrive when nourished by a nutrient-rich diet.

You can help prime your child's brain cells for optimal learning by focusing on two key nutrients essential for healthy cell membranes not only in the brain, but throughout the body. These nutrients are choline and omega-3 essential fatty acids.

Choline

Choline is a chemical cousin to the vitamin B family. It serves as a building block for phosphatidylcholine, sometimes referred to as lecithin. This fat-like compound wiggles its way into the membranes that surround brain cells and other cells where it not only fortifies the structural integrity of the membrane, which helps control the flow of materials into and out of the cell, but also plays quarterback in the chemical signaling that triggers cells into action.

The body also uses choline to synthesize acetylcholine, a chemical messenger in the brain that's critical for cell-to-cell communication involved in learning, memory and other functions. Nutrition experts recommend that younger children, aged 4 to 8 years, consume at least 250 milligrams of choline per day, but avoid exceeding 1,000 milligrams per day. Older kids, aged 9 to 13 years, should consume at least 375 milligrams of choline per day, but avoid exceeding 2,000 milligrams per day.

Food sources of choline

What foods are good sources of choline? It's widely distributed in foods, but the most common kid-friendly foods are milk and egg yolks. Each cup of milk provides about 40 milligrams of choline, and each egg provides at least 100 milligrams of choline. But don't overlook other sources of choline that your child may enjoy such as foods made with soybeans, beef, fish, chicken, peanuts or vegetables such as cauliflower and cabbage.

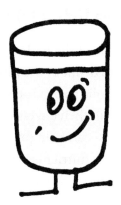

Omega-3 Fatty Acids

Omega-3 fatty acids are among the largest fatty acids found in the body. They are often called long-chain fatty acids because they sit on chemical backbones ranging from 18 to 22 carbon molecules—Goliath in biochemical terms.

When it comes to brain health, two omega-3 fatty acids—ALA (alpha-linolenic acid) and EPA (eicosapentaenoic acid)—can lend a helping hand, but the star is DHA (docosahexaenoic acid). We must consume ALA in the foods we eat because our bodies can't make it. But after we consume ALA, our bodies can summon a few enzymes into action to convert it into EPA and finally into DHA. Why is this conversion so important? Both EPA and DHA influence the physical nature of cell membranes and cellular functions, while DHA plays an important structural role in the eye and brain. Trouble is, the rate of conversion is less than impressive. In fact, some researchers report that the body converts only about 15 percent of the typical ALA intake to EPA and DHA.

According to Barry Sears, Ph.D., author of *The Omega Rx Zone*, "Trying to maintain brain function without adequate DHA is like trying to build the sturdiest brick house in town without enough bricks. You might have the best architect, the best location, and the best contractor, but if you don't have enough bricks, the dream house will never be built properly. Without adequate DHA, your brain can't function adequately and can't form new neuronal connections, let alone maintain old ones."

Now, we don't have to rely on the body to convert ALA to DHA if we eat enough DHA-rich foods, but sadly, the typical American diet doesn't come close to providing an adequate intake. For example, health experts recommend a daily intake of at least 650 milligrams for EPA and DHA combined. Yet, researchers report the typical American diet provides only about one-third of this amount—about 100 to 200 milligrams per day.

Food sources of omega-3 fats

What foods are good sources of omega-3 fatty acids? English walnuts, flaxseed, green leafy vegetables such as purslane and spinach and certain vegetable oils—canola, soybean, flaxseed, linseed and olive—are particularly good sources of ALA. The only foods that supply substantial amounts of EPA and DHA are fish—particularly cold-water fish such as salmon, haddock, mackerel, tuna, anchovies and sardines.

Fish oils are also a good source of EPA and DHA, and manufacturers are adding these brain-boosting fats to a wide variety of packaged foods such as orange juice and eggs. So, it's worth taking the time to compare labels to choose a brand fortified with omega-3's.

Parent Pearl

I give my kids a fish oil supplement every day. It helps ensure they're getting enough brain-building omega-3 DHA. To entice them, I buy a brand that offers the DHA in a gumdrop-type delivery system.

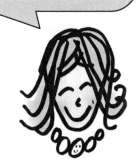

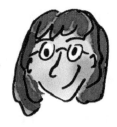

Did You Know?

Walnuts, flaxseed and certain vegetable oils are some of the richest food sources of ALA. Cold-water fish such as salmon, tuna and others are one of the best food sources of EPA and DHA.

Food	Omega-3 Fatty Acid (milligrams)	
	ALA	EPA + DHA
Walnuts, English (14 halves)	2,600 mg	--
Flaxseed oil (1 teaspoon)	2,400 mg	--
Flaxseed, ground (1 teaspoon)	600 mg	--
Canola oil (1 teaspoon)	430 mg	--
Soybean oil (1 teaspoon)	230 mg	--
Spinach, cooked (½ cup)	80 mg	--
Olive oil (1 teaspoon)	30 mg	--
Tuna, canned in water (3 ounces)	60 mg	700 mg
Salmon, cooked (3 ounces)	40 mg	700 mg
Sardines, canned in oil (2 each)	100 mg	200 mg

Source: USDA Nutrient Database.

A word of caution

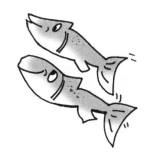

While fish is a great source of DHA, the brain-boosting omega-3 fatty acid, some types—shark, swordfish, king mackerel and tilefish—tend to concentrate higher amounts of the toxic heavy metal mercury. What's a parent to do? Choose fish that are known to be lower in mercury more often. Think shellfish, canned fish, smaller ocean fish and farm-raised fish. Or, consider supplementing with fish oil, which contains less mercury compared to fish meat. High-quality fish oil supplements meet strict standards to ensure low mercury content.

High-Octane Foods

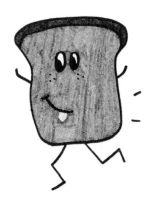

When it comes to fueling your child's brain for focused attention and learning, nothing beats starchy foods. Nutrition experts call these complex carbohydrates. You can call them high-octane fuel for growing brains. Your best bets are starchy foods that are also high in fiber. Think whole grain cereals, breads and pastas as well as brown rice, peas, beans and starchy veggies.

From the first bite, these foods set off a cascade of digestive enzymes that go to work breaking down large starch molecules into simple sugars that the body is able to absorb and release into the bloodstream to fuel organs and tissues. One such simple sugar, glucose, is the brain's main energy source.

As the body's most complex organ, the brain demands an enormous amount of energy and requires constant refueling. How do you ensure your child's brain has a steady supply of glucose for learning? It all has to do with keeping the blood glucose level fairly steady throughout the day—not too much and not too little. Some starchy foods work better than others at this. These are the so-called low-GI foods.

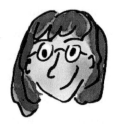

Did You Know?

Foods made with whole grains use the entire grain seed so they provide all the naturally occurring nutrients. Here's a list of common—and not so common—whole grains to look for in foods:

Barley	Millet	Sorghum
Brown rice	Oats	Triticale
Buckwheat	Quinoa	Wheat
Bulgur	Rye	Wild rice
Corn		

For a complete list of whole grain foods, visit www.wholegrainscouncil.org.

GI or glycemic index is a system for ranking foods based on how they affect blood glucose levels immediately after being consumed. Carbohydrates that are digested slowly have lower GI values. They release glucose into the bloodstream gradually, drip by drip, which helps maintain a steady blood level after you eat them. Examples include an orange, whole wheat bread and oatmeal.

By contrast, carbohydrates that are digested quickly—white bread, white rice, potatoes and the like—have higher GI values. These foods are absorbed into the body quickly and flood the bloodstream leading to a blood sugar response that can be too fast and too high.

What's the best way to use the GI system for brain health? It's easy. No need to banish high-GI foods from the diet, just choose them less often or balance them with low-GI foods at the same meal. Whenever possible, serve up low-GI options of your favorite carb-rich foods—a bowl of stick-to-your-ribs porridge made with rolled oats rather than a plain bagel for breakfast; whole wheat bread instead of white bread for a lunchbox sandwich; or nutty brown rice instead of plain white rice at dinner.

Parent Pearl

My kids can be finicky when it comes to eating broccoli and other steamed veggies. So, I garnish with just enough grated cheese for flavor—about 1 teaspoon per serving. It's a delicious, nutrient-rich way to boost their veggie intake.

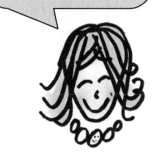

To find the GI value of your favorite foods, visit www.glycemicindex.com. Here, you'll find a searchable database of foods based on their GI value. Including foods with a low GI value—55 or less—at meals and snacks will help ensure healthy blood glucose levels after eating. It's an ideal way to help refuel busy brains with energizing glucose from the first morning class to long after homework is done.

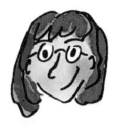

Did You Know?

When consumed alone, foods with a high Glycemic Index (GI)—55 or above—can lead to a blood sugar response that can be too fast and too high. You don't have to avoid high GI foods for better blood glucose control. Simply consume them with foods that have a lower GI value at the same meal or snack. Remember, only foods that contain carbohydrates have a GI value. Meat, fish, eggs, avocado and other foods containing little or no carbs can't have a GI value. In short: No carbs, no GI value.

Food	GI Value*	GI Rank
Potato, white, without skin	98	High
Rice, white, long grain	76	High
Bread, white	75	High
Bagel, white bread	69	High
Bread, whole wheat	52	Low
Rice, brown	50	Low
Porridge, rolled oats	42	Low
Orange	33	Low

* Representative sample. Source: www.glycemicindex.com.

This Month's Smart Goal

I will serve breakfast every day and include a protein-rich food.

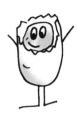

This Month's Extra Credit

I will give my child a DHA supplement every day, preferably at breakfast.

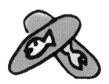

To monitor your daily progress toward your goals, use the **My Smart Tracker** forms in Chapter 14: Go for the Goal!

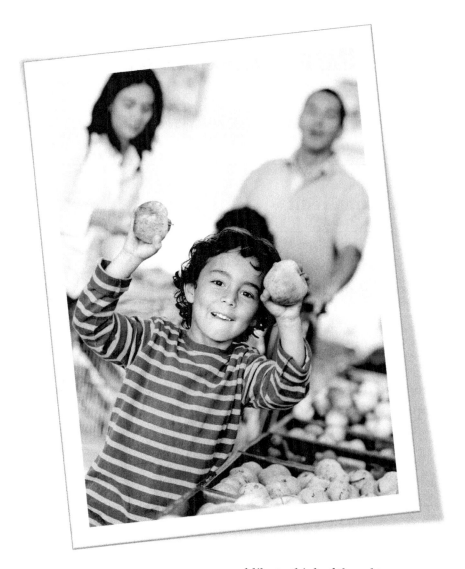

I like to think of thoughts as
living blossoms borne by the human tree.
– James Douglas

Chapter 4

November – Eat Your Colors

Mother Nature surrounds us with beautiful colors all year round. Think of green leaves transforming into brilliant reds, oranges and yellows as summer fades into autumn, or imagine a rainbow bursting forth after a spring shower. Fruits and vegetables are no exception with a rich color palette—deep purple plums, vibrant red peppers, sunny oranges, crisp green lettuce, white cauliflower—in just about every hue imaginable.

Like many parents, you may not think twice about the color of the fruits and vegetables you feed your child. Yet, helping your child eat a diet rich in colorful fruits and veggies can have a profound impact on overall health, including brain health. In fact, this simple behavior—eating a wide variety of colors—is one of the most significant dietary habits that you can establish to steer your child toward a healthier future while promoting brain health and protecting brain cells from damage.

Why should you focus on serving up meals in living color? In a word: Phytonutrients. Plants produce a wide variety of these bioactive compounds as protection against a whole host of environmental insults from insect infestations to extreme temperatures to pesticide exposure, just to name a few. When your child eats them, these very same phytonutrients go to work to protect overall health, including brain health.

What's the best way to ensure that your child is eating the amount and type of phytonutrients that will protect their brain? Make sure they eat a colorful diet. How? Simply focus on eating fruits and veggies with skin or flesh in the five key color groups—purple, red, orange-yellow, green and white—every day. The good news is it's easier than you may think, especially after a quick primer on each of these colorful food groups. Read on to get started.

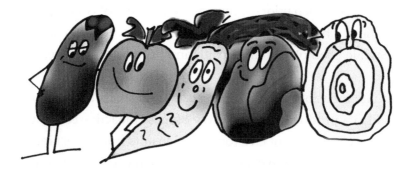

The Purple Group

Purple fruits and vegetables come in a variety of shades from the deep violet purple of an eggplant to the purple-red of a beet to the bluish purple of blueberries. These fruits and vegetables tend to be rich sources of anthocyanins, a group of phytonutrients shown to promote brain health.

How do anthocyanins work in the body? Anthocyanins are powerful antioxidants, as well as anti-inflammatory agents. In the brain and throughout the body, antioxidants help protect cells from the so-called "free radicals" that result from normal cellular metabolism. When the brain is unable to neutralize these unstable biochemical byproducts, oxidative stress can occur that can damage and destroy healthy brain cells. A well-nourished brain, by contrast, is primed to neutralize destructive free radicals thanks to a diet rich in antioxidants, including brain-boosting anthocyanins. You'll learn more about the importance of antioxidants in Chapter 5: December – De-Stress, Sleep & Learn.

The "Brainberry"

One of the stars of the purple group is the blueberry, which is both kid-friendly and brimming with protective antioxidants. This tiny berry packs some mighty brain benefits earning it the prestigious nickname "brainberry."

In 1999, James Joseph, Ph.D., and his colleagues at Tufts University were among the first to report

Parent Pearl

Soup for the soul.
When the weather starts to cool down, I find the best way to warm up my family is with a bowl of homemade soup. A simmering kettle of fresh vegetable soup coupled with a crusty whole grain roll makes for a wonderful and nourishing dinner.

the brain benefits of blueberries and other berries in laboratory rats. Publishing their findings in the *Journal of Neuroscience*, the researchers found that rats fed the equivalent of 1 cup of blueberries each day for two months actually improved their short-term memory.

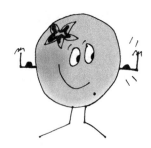

How does your child's intake of fruits and vegetables in the purple group rate? Take our **Purple Power Assessment** to find out.

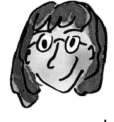

Did You Know?

The USDA's Center for Nutrition Policy and Promotion offers a great online resource for fun facts and activities to inspire your kids to eat more fruits and vegetables. Visit www.choosemyplate.gov.

Here you'll find coloring sheets, worksheets and other fun paper-and-pencil activities. For computer lovers, there's even an interactive computer game, Blast Off, where kids can choose fruits, veggies and other foods along with activity to fuel their rocket to reach Planet Power. Make it a family affair—get everyone involved.

Purple Power Assessment

Check (☑) the box for each food below that your child eats. Enter the total number of foods at the bottom. Read on to learn how your child's diet rates.

- ❑ Beets
- ❑ Blackberries
- ❑ Blueberries
- ❑ Boysenberries
- ❑ Cabbage (red)
- ❑ Cherries
- ❑ Other:_____

- ❑ Currants (black)
- ❑ Eggplant
- ❑ Elderberries
- ❑ Figs (purple)
- ❑ Grapes (Concord)
- ❑ Huckleberries

- ❑ Ollalieberries
- ❑ Plum
- ❑ Potato (purple)
- ❑ Prunes
- ❑ Raisins
- ❑ Rhubarb

Enter the total number here.

How Did Your Child Do?

If your child currently consumes more than 10 different purple fruits and vegetables, you both deserve a big pat on the back. Bravo! If not, consider adding one or two more purple fruits or vegetables to your family's diet this month. Make it a fun adventure as you shop for these purple beauties at your local grocery or farmers market. Don't forget the frozen section, where out-of-season produce such as blueberries, can be found year round.

The Red Group

Some red foods get their color from lycopene, a key phytonutrient with powerful antioxidant activity.

Researchers are discovering that this natural plant compound helps promote heart and circulatory health. That's good news for an active brain as a healthy circulation means blood can carry nutrients to your child's brain and whisk away metabolic waste with ease. What's more, a well-nourished brain is one that can function at peak performance.

Like the purple food group, some fruits and vegetables in the red group contain anthocyanins with antioxidant and anti-inflammatory properties.

So, how does your child's intake of red fruits and vegetables rate? Take our **Red Rocks Assessment** to find out.

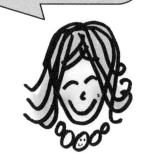

Parent Pearl

Consider adding pomegranate seeds to your child's diet. We do this at home and they are a true crowd pleaser. Just make sure you have plenty of napkins!

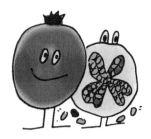

Red Rocks Assessment

Check (☑) the box for each food below that your child eats. Enter the total number of foods at the bottom. Read on to learn how your child's diet rates.

- ❑ Apple (red)†
- ❑ Chokeberries†
- ❑ Cranberries†
- ❑ Grapefruit (pink, red)*
- ❑ Grapes (red)†
- ❑ Kidney beans (red)†
- ❑ Lettuce (red)†
- ❑ Mango†
- ❑ Onion (red)†
- ❑ Papaya (pink)*
- ❑ Pepper (sweet)*
- ❑ Pomegranate†
- ❑ Radishes†
- ❑ Raspberries†
- ❑ Red currants†
- ❑ Strawberries†
- ❑ Tomato (including tomato paste, ketchup and spaghetti sauce)*
- ❑ Watermelon*

- ❑ Other:_____

* rich in lycopene

† rich in anthocyanins

Enter the total number here.

How Did Your Child Do?

If your child currently consumes more than 10 different red fruits and vegetables, excellent! If not, consider adding one or two more to your family's diet this month. In this case, even ketchup and spaghetti sauce count because they're loaded with lycopene.

The Orange-Yellow Group

Fruits and vegetables in the orange-yellow group tend to be rich in phytonutrients known as carotenoids such as alpha-carotene, beta-carotene, beta-cryptoxanthin, lutein and zeaxanthin.

Fruits and vegetables with these brain-protecting antioxidants are also being studied for their potential benefits for heart and immune health and healthy vision.

How does your child's diet rate in terms of these orange-yellow beauties? Take our **Outrageous Orange-Yellow Assessment** to find out.

Parent Pearl

Show them they're a star! My kids love the exotic carambola fruit. To make this yellow-orange fruit extra special, I slice crosswise and serve up the natural star-shaped slices. It's a delicious way to boost nutrition.

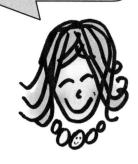

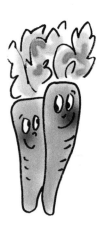

Outrageous Orange-Yellow Assessment

> Check (☑) the box for each food below that your child eats. Enter the total number of foods at the bottom. Read on to learn how your child's diet rates.

- ❑ Apricots*
- ❑ Bell pepper (yellow)*
- ❑ Cantaloupe*
- ❑ Cape gooseberries
- ❑ Carambola*
- ❑ Carrot*
- ❑ Corn*
- ❑ Kumquats

- ❑ Lemon
- ❑ Mango*
- ❑ Melon (casaba, Crenshaw, Persian)
- ❑ Nectarine
- ❑ Orange
- ❑ Papaya
- ❑ Passion fruit
- ❑ Peach

- ❑ Pear (golden)
- ❑ Persimmon*
- ❑ Pineapple
- ❑ Plantain
- ❑ Potato (yellow)
- ❑ Pumpkin*
- ❑ Quince
- ❑ Tangelo

- ❑ Tangerine*
- ❑ Rutabaga
- ❑ Summer squash (yellow)*
- ❑ Sweet potato*
- ❑ Winter squash (acorn, banana, butternut, spaghetti)*
- ❑ Yam*

Other:_____

* rich in alpha-carotene, beta-carotene, lutein or zeaxanthin

☐ Enter the total number here.

How Did Your Child Do?

If your child's diet includes 15 or more fruits and vegetables in the orange-yellow color group, great job! If your child's diet includes between eight and 10 of these carotenoid-rich beauties, it's still a job well done. For more variety, consider adding another orange-yellow fruits or veggies to your child's diet each week until your child is enjoying a wider variety of these protective foods. If no more than seven foods are showing up in your child's diet, it's time to focus. Pull out the cookbooks, and use your creative juices. You may be surprised at the results.

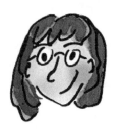

Did You Know?

A wealth of expert advice on fruits and veggies is a click away at www.fruitsandveggiesmorematters.org.

Here you'll find a library of fun facts, practical planning, shopping and cooking tips, kid-friendly activities and much more—all focused on inspiring kids and adults alike to eat more fruits, veggies and nuts.

The Green Group

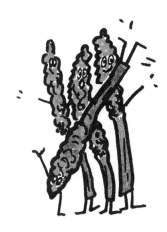

Fruits and vegetables in the green group contain a wide variety of beneficial phytonutrients. For example, vegetables in the cruciferous family such as broccoli, kale, collard greens and bok choy are natural sources of sulforaphane, isothiocyanates, indoles and other phytonutrients with tongue-twister names.

These plant powerhouses rev up the liver's production of enzymes that help keep cells throughout the body healthy.

How does your child's intake of fruits and vegetables in the green group rate? Take our **Go Green Assessment** on page 65 to find out.

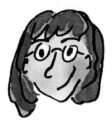

Did You Know?

You can encourage your child to be an artist when it comes to selecting fruits and vegetables. Think of it as painting a rainbow on the plate using as many of the color groups as possible—red, orange-yellow, green, purple-blue and white. The more colors, the better for your child's health.

As a general rule, have your child strive to include at least three natural colors on their plate at meal times. Make it a game; see who can design the most colorful platter.

Go Green Assessment

Check (☑) the box for each food below that your child eats. Enter the total number of foods at the bottom. Read on to learn how your child's diet rates.

- ❑ Apple (green)
- ❑ Artichoke
- ❑ Arugula
- ❑ Asparagus
- ❑ Avocado
- ❑ Bell pepper (green)
- ❑ Bok choy*
- ❑ Broccoli*
- ❑ Brussels sprouts*
- ❑ Cabbage (green)
- ❑ Cactus
- ❑ Celery

- ❑ Collard greens*
- ❑ Cucumber
- ❑ Fennel
- ❑ Grapes (green)
- ❑ Green beans
- ❑ Honeydew melon
- ❑ Kale*
- ❑ Kiwi
- ❑ Leek
- ❑ Lettuce (butter, iceberg, romaine, etc.)
- ❑ Lima beans

- ❑ Lime
- ❑ Mustard greens*
- ❑ Okra
- ❑ Onion (green)
- ❑ Pear (green)
- ❑ Peas
- ❑ Spinach
- ❑ Swiss chard*
- ❑ Turnip green
- ❑ Watercress
- ❑ Wax beans
- ❑ Zucchini

- ❑ Other:_____

* rich in isothiocyanates or indoles

| | Enter the total number here.

How Did Your Child Do?

If your child's diet includes 20 or more fruits and vegetables in the green color group, we would like to give you a standing ovation. Great job! If your child's diet includes between eight and 19 greens, we'd give you a B+! If you squeaked out no more than seven greens, it's time to revisit the list of foods to select more. The good news is, with so many kid-friendly greens to choose from, it's relatively easy to add a few more to your child's diet.

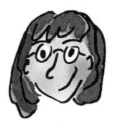

Did You Know?

The phytonutrients in different colored fruits and veggies deliver distinct health benefits. Ask your child to study a fruit or vegetable and describe what they see—the star on a blueberry or the golden-red splotches on a peach. Remind your child that each color works in its own special way to protect both body and brain.

The White Group

Just because white fruits and vegetables are pale, doesn't mean they don't pack a nutritious punch. Onion, garlic, chive, leek, shallots and other pale members of the allium family contain allicin, a naturally occurring antioxidant that also promotes circulatory health and boosts the immune system. Some white foods such as onion, garlic and apple are also a natural source of quercetin, a phytonutrient with anti-inflammatory properties.

How does your child's intake of fruits and vegetables in the white group rate? Take our **Wonderful White Assessment** on page 68 to find out.

Parent Pearl

For an exotic treat, I serve cherimoya. With white flesh and black almond-shaped seeds, this fruit has a texture like custard but tastes like a combination of banana, pineapple and papaya. And, it's a good source of vitamin C and fiber. The kids love it, especially when chilled.

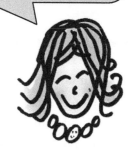

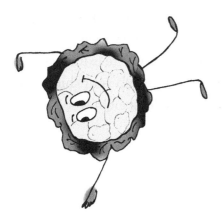

Wonderful White Assessment

> Check (☑) the box for each food below that your child eats. Enter the total number of foods at the bottom. Read on to see how your child's diet rates.

❑ Banana   ❑ Cherimoya   ❑ Jicama   ❑ Pinto beans†

❑ Belgian endive   ❑ Chestnuts   ❑ Kohlrabi   ❑ Potato (russet)

❑ Black beans†   ❑ Chives*   ❑ Leek*   ❑ Radishes

❑ Broccoflower   ❑ Coconut   ❑ Morels   ❑ Rutabaga

❑ Cauliflower   ❑ Dates†   ❑ Mushrooms   ❑ Shallots*

❑ Celery root   ❑ Garlic*   ❑ Onion (white)*   ❑ Turnip

❑ Chayote squash   ❑ Ginger   ❑ Parsnip

❑ Other:_____

* rich in allicin

† while not white in color, don't forget these nutritional wonders

[   ] Enter the total number here.

How Did Your Child Do?

If your child's diet includes 15 or more fruits and vegetables in the white color group, you're really a superstar—this is one of the tougher groups from which to choose a wide variety. If your child's diet includes between eight and 14 whites, give yourself a pat on the back, but don't forget to work on boosting the variety.

If your child's diet has fewer than seven white foods, this is where extra focus will pay off. Consider incorporating a new white fruit or veggie into your child's diet this week. Continue each week until your child is enjoying at least eight wonderful whites on a regular basis.

Active Brains Benefit from Variety

When it comes to choosing fruits and veggies to include in your child's diet, the more variety, the better. Why? Each color group delivers its own specific health benefits to promote brain health, protect brain cells from oxidative stress and support optimal health. So, top on your list of brain-boosting goals should be including a wide range of richly colored fruits and vegetables on your child's plate— every day. What's more, focusing on including a variety of colorful fruits and vegetables in your child's diet will also help ensure their intake is adequate for overall health.

Unfortunately, most children fail to achieve this goal so they miss out on both the body and brain benefits. For example, according to the Third National Health and Nutrition Examination Survey sponsored by the U.S. Department of Agriculture, four out of five elementary school-aged children fail to eat the recommended five or more servings of fruits and vegetables each day. And, the average 6- to 11-year-old eats only three and one-half servings. Finally, on any given day, more than half of all elementary school-age children eat no fruit and three out of 10 eat fewer than one serving of vegetables.

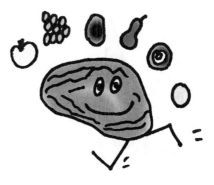

How Much Should Your Child Eat?

Experts recommend children eat at least 3 to 5 cups of fruits and vegetables every day, depending on their grade level and age. The chart below provides a quick reference guide. However, when it comes to consuming fruits and vegetables, the general rule is: The more, the better!

Recommended Daily Fruit and Vegetable Intake for Elementary School-Aged Children*		
Grade (Age)	**Fruits**	**Vegetables**
Kindergarten (5 to 6 years)	1½ cups	1½ cups
First Grade (6 to 7 years)	1½ cups	1½ to 2 cups
Second Grade (7 to 8 years)	1½ cups	2 cups
Third Grade (8 to 9 years)	1½ cups	2 to 2½ cups
Fourth Grade (9 to 10 years)	1½ cups	2 to 2½ cups
Fifth Grade (10 to 11 years)	1½ to 2 cups	2½ cups
Sixth Grade (11 to 12 years)	1½ to 2 cups	2½ to 3 cups
* For a moderately active child (30-60 minutes of activity per day).		

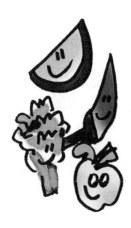

Six Easy Steps to More Fruits & Veggies

1 **Keep fruits and vegetables visible.** Fill a fruit bowl and put it in an easily accessible spot in your kitchen, or place a tray full of ready-to-munch raw vegetables in the refrigerator at your child's eye level. According to Brian Wansink, Ph.D., the typical person will make over 200 food-related decisions daily. What's more, Dr. Wansink notes that we don't even think about nine out of 10 of those decisions. That's right, most of our food-related decisions are subconscious. This suggests that it may be much easier to control your environment than to control your willpower. If so, why not start with the one

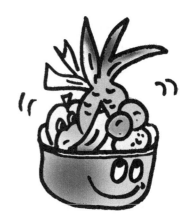

environment that you can control the most: Your home. Stock your pantry with lots of healthy food choices prepared for easy munching so your child has plenty of opportunity to nourish his or her growing body and brain. For more information, see **Stocking Your Fridge, Freezer & Pantry** in Chapter 15: Tables, Tips & More.

2 **Let them munch while you make meals.** Offer veggies as you prepare the family meal—carrot sticks, jicama slices or other crunchy favorites take only a few extra minutes to prepare once you're in food prep mode for the meal. Talk about a simple solution. You may be surprised at how much your child will gobble up!

3 **Slip in extra helpings of veggies and fruits.** Consider adding finely chopped carrots, eggplant, broccoli, cauliflower or other veggies to marinara sauce, soups, stews and chili. Try stuffing a pita pocket with veggie chunks or offering a fruit salad or smoothie as a snack or dessert.

4 **Try roasting vegetables for a deep, rich flavor.**
Drizzle veggies with a little olive oil and roast in an oven set to 425 degrees Fahrenheit or on the grill until tender. Try carrots, asparagus, butternut squash, eggplant, broccoli or just about any vegetable that you like.

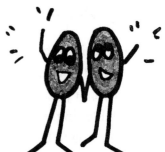

5 **Pack and go.** Toss snap peas, soybeans, carrots, jicama, baby tomatoes or other pieces of raw vegetables in a plastic bag for your child to munch on when away from home.

6 **Let them choose.** When grocery shopping, allow your child to select a fruit or vegetable that he or she wants to eat.

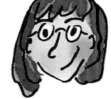

Did You Know?

When adding more fruits and vegetables into your child's diet, think local and seasonal. To find out what's growing in your local area, visit Local Harvest (www.localharvest.org), which provides a nationwide directory of small farms, farmers markets and other local food sources.

Organic: Is It Really Better?

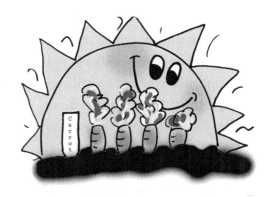

Are organically grown fruits and vegetables more nutritious? The jury is still out. There are only a few well-controlled studies comparing the nutrient content of organic and conventionally grown fruits and vegetables. In general, these studies fail to show a significant difference in the amounts of micronutrients such as vitamins, minerals and trace elements. However, there appears to be a slight trend toward higher vitamin C content in organically grown leafy vegetables and potatoes.

Are organic foods tastier? Some folks say that organic foods taste much better than conventionally grown foods. Others say that there is no difference. Since taste is a subjective matter, only you would be the best judge. Whether you decide to buy foods that are grown organically or conventionally, choosing the freshest foods available is likely to have the biggest impact on taste. If possible, choose locally grown foods as these tend to be the freshest.

Are organic foods safer? According to a recent study published in the scientific journal *Environmental Health Perspectives*, Dr. Chensheng Lu and colleagues at Emory University found the amount of toxic pesticides in children's bodies was dramatically and immediately lowered after they switched from a diet with conventionally grown foods to one with organic foods. The researchers followed 23 elementary school-aged children for 15 days. On five of those days, the children were given organic produce, juice, grains and other organic foods. After only five days on the organic diet, the level of organophosphorus pesticides found in the children's urine plummeted to undetectable levels.

Should you be worried? Although conventionally grown produce contains higher levels of pesticide residues, it does not necessarily mean that they are dangerous to your child's health. The level of pesticides in children's urine has not been definitively linked to any health problems. However, it would be difficult to refute that reducing overall pesticide exposure offers some health benefits.

According to Dr. Lu and study co-author Dr. Richard Fenske, the health risks to children are still uncertain. However, Dr. Lu points out that there is no getting around the fact that a pesticide is a neurotoxin. Since pesticides disrupt enzymes in the brain critical for cell-to-cell communication, exposing your child to pesticides could potentially damage the brain. These chemicals are developed, after all, to kill bugs by paralyzing or over-exciting their nervous systems.

An Easy Way to Avoid Pesticides

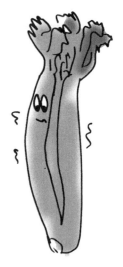

The amount of pesticide residue in fruits and vegetables varies, but you can help keep your child's exposure to a minimum by choosing wisely from the "Dirty Dozen" and "Clean 15" lists of fruits and vegetables.

What are these lists? They are based on a report published by the Environmental Working Group (EWG). The 12 fruits and vegetables that consistently have the highest levels of pesticides have been dubbed the "Dirty Dozen," with celery topping the list. To come up with its rankings, the EWG examined the results of nearly 96,000 tests for pesticides on produce performed by the USDA and the U.S. Food and Drug Administration. Conversely, the "Clean 15" list represents those fruits and vegetables with the lowest pesticide residue.

If your child's favorites are among the Dirty Dozen, buy organic whenever possible. If you don't see your child's favorites, visit www.foodnews.org for additional information and the most recent test results.

The "Dirty Dozen"
(Highest in Pesticide Residue)

1. Celery
2. Peach
3. Strawberries
4. Apple
5. Blueberries
6. Nectarine
7. Bell pepper
8. Spinach
9. Kale
10. Cherries
11. Potato
12. Grapes (imported)

The "Clean 15"
(Lowest in Pesticide Residue)

1. Onion
2. Avocado
3. Sweet corn
4. Pineapple
5. Mango
6. Sweet peas
7. Asparagus
8. Kiwi
9. Cabbage
10. Eggplant
11. Cantaloupe
12. Watermelon
13. Grapefruit
14. Sweet potato
15. Honeydew melon

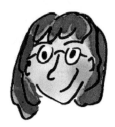

Did You Know?

You can easily find a registered dietitian in your area who specializes in child nutrition. Ask your pediatrician or visit the Academy of Nutrition and Dietetics website at www.eatright.org. Click on "Find a Registered Dietitian" to access a national database of qualified nutrition experts that is searchable by both expertise and location.

Healthy Choices for Every Budget

In general, organic foods are more expensive than conventional foods. But, you don't need to choose 100 percent organic fruits and vegetables to get protective benefits. With four simple food shopping and preparation tips, you can make healthier choices—and remain budget-conscious. Here's how:

1 **Review the "Dirty Dozen" list.** If your child's favorites are on the list, focus on buying those foods organically grown.

2 **Wash and peel.** Wash fruits and vegetables thoroughly. If you're concerned about pesticides, peel your fruits and vegetables and trim outer leaves of leafy vegetables.

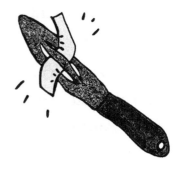

3 **Encourage variety.** This will help avoid eating one particular fruit or vegetable that may contain high levels of pesticides. Variety also helps supply more protective phytonutrients and nourishing vitamins and minerals.

4 **Look at the big picture.** If your child's diet is full of processed and fast foods, it's best to begin by making more general lifestyle changes such as having them eat more fruits and vegetables, legumes and whole grains—whether they are organic or not—and eat less processed, refined and fast foods. When this becomes a regular habit, then consider exploring organic options. Remember, it's not a race to good nutrition. It's a step-by-step, one-day-at-a-time process that leads to a lifetime of healthful eating. Your child will get there.

This Month's Smart Goal

I will add ½ cup of fruits or vegetables each week until my child meets the recommended intake (at least 3 to 5 cups daily based on age).

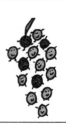

This Month's Extra Credit

I will serve a fruit or veggie in each color group (purple, red, orange-yellow, green and white) at least three days per week.

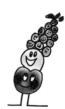

To monitor your daily progress toward your goals, use the **My Smart Tracker** forms in Chapter 14: Go for the Goal!

Part 3
Winter Season

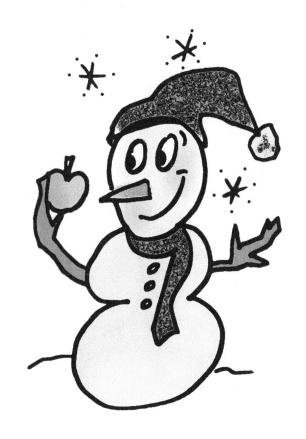

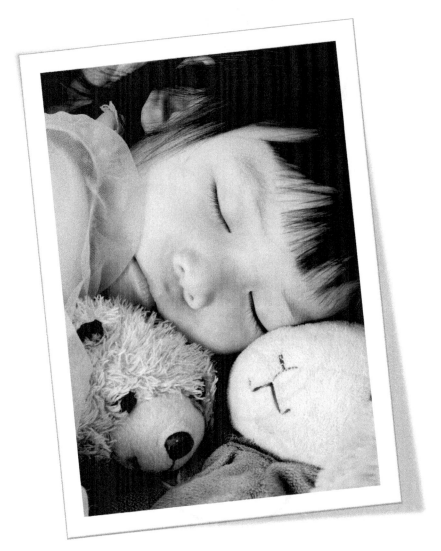

Brain cells create ideas.
Stress kills brain cells.
Stress is not a good idea.
    — Frederick Saunders

Chapter 5

December – De-Stress, Sleep & Learn

Your child's brain is a flurry of non-stop activity whether it's called into action for brushing teeth, singing a favorite song or preparing for a classroom quiz. Even when your rising star is snoozing, brain cells remain active processing the day's events and shuttling information into long-term memory.

All this hard work requires constant refueling with energy, nutrients and oxygen not only to survive, but to flourish and grow. In fact, for an organ that makes up a trivial 2 percent of body weight, the brain uses a whopping 20 percent of the oxygen breathed in. With the number of brain cells estimated to be in the billions and beyond, this translates into an enormous amount of biochemical action.

Brain cells drink in oxygen to fuel the cell-to-cell communication critical for learning and memory. The trouble is, the process isn't quite perfect. All this constant biochemical activity tends to produce metabolic byproducts that can actually harm brain cells. Scientists call these molecules reactive oxygen species, and you may know them as free radicals. Either way, these unstable molecules cause oxidative stress, which can wreak havoc with brain cells and even cause cell death.

Your Best Strategy

What's the best strategy to protect your child's brain against potential free radical damage? The most powerful first line of defense is a healthy diet, rich in antioxidants. These biochemical wonders trap free radicals before they can damage brain cells. So, ensuring your child consumes lots of antioxidant-rich foods is essential for brain health.

ORAC Value

How do you know which foods are bursting with antioxidant protection and which are just so-so? One way is to compare foods based on their ORAC value. ORAC stands for Oxygen Radical Absorbance Capacity, which is a high-tech laboratory test that researchers use to measure a food's antioxidant power. In fact, researchers at the U.S. Department of Agriculture have now measured the ORAC value of over 120 fruits, vegetables, nuts, spices and herbs.

Star Power Foods

We've selected the best choices from their research to bring you **Star Power Foods**—a list of common fruits, vegetables, nuts and spices that are both antioxidant-rich and kid-friendly. Are these brain foods in your child's diet? Read on to find out.

> ### Parent Pearl
>
> **We use fun mnemonics and other memory aids to remember new information.** My favorite is a catchy aide to remember the order of the planets: "My very eager mother just served us nine pizzas!"
>
> | | |
> |---|---|
> | Mercury | (my) |
> | Venus | (very) |
> | Earth | (eager) |
> | Mars | (mother) |
> | Jupiter | (just) |
> | Saturn | (served) |
> | Uranus | (us) |
> | Neptune | (nine) |
> | Pluto | (pizzas) |

Star Power Foods

Check (☑) the box for each antioxidant-rich food in your child's diet.
More is better!

BEST

- ❏ Artichoke
- ❏ Blackberries
- ❏ Blueberries

- ❏ Cranberries
- ❏ Kidney beans

- ❏ Pinto beans
- ❏ Red beans

BETTER

- ❏ Apple
- ❏ Avocado
- ❏ Black beans
- ❏ Cherries

- ❏ Dates (Deglet Noor)
- ❏ Pecans
- ❏ Plum
- ❏ Potato (red, russet)

- ❏ Prunes
- ❏ Raspberries
- ❏ Strawberries
- ❏ Walnuts

GOOD

- ❏ Almonds
- ❏ Apricots
- ❏ Asparagus
- ❏ Beet
- ❏ Blackeye peas
- ❏ Broccoli
- ❏ Cabbage (red)
- ❏ Cinnamon
- ❏ Clove
- ❏ Dates (Medjool)
- ❏ Figs
- ❏ Grapefruit (red)

- ❏ Grapes
- ❏ Hazelnuts
- ❏ Lettuce (red)
- ❏ Mango
- ❏ Navy beans
- ❏ Onion
- ❏ Orange (navel)
- ❏ Oregano
- ❏ Peach
- ❏ Pear
- ❏ Pineapple
- ❏ Pistachios

- ❏ Potato (white)
- ❏ Radish
- ❏ Raisins
- ❏ Sweet pepper
- ❏ Sweet potato
- ❏ Tangerine
- ❏ Turmeric

4 Steps to Boost Antioxidant Intake

Helping your child consume a rich supply of antioxidants for brain health and optimal learning may be easier than you think. Read on for an easy four-step strategy that you can begin today.

1 **Build on your child's favorites.** It's a good bet that antioxidant-rich foods are already among your child's favorites, and others could easily become new favorites. For a quick check, take a look at the list of **Star Power Foods** on page 83. Serving these foods on a regular basis will help ensure your child obtains the antioxidant protection that an active brain needs.

2 **Make small changes to every meal.** Include at least one antioxidant-rich food at every meal. Not only will this help bathe the brain in protective antioxidants throughout the day, but it's sure to help shape a life-long habit of eating these nutritious foods on a regular basis.

3 **Add variety.** When it comes to antioxidant support, the more variety, the better. Why? Plant foods naturally contain a wide array of bioactive compounds with antioxidant properties that can help shield growing brains—and bodies—from the harmful effects of oxygen free radicals. You can't beat fruits and vegetables to boost antioxidant intake, but don't forget about nuts, spices and herbs, which offer antioxidant benefits as well. With a few smart choices, you'll have plenty of opportunity to include the protective power of antioxidants in meals and snacks for your kids.

Parent Pearl

I fill an extra salt shaker with cinnamon and keep it handy. It's an easy solution to bring this favorite antioxidant-rich spice out of the cupboard and onto the table. This tasty topping is great for hot chocolate, oatmeal, toast, applesauce and so many more of my kid's favorite foods.

4 **Consider extra protection for today's lifestyles.** The body's production of harmful free radicals can ramp up under certain circumstances. This holds true for kids and adults alike. In these situations, extra antioxidant protection can be especially helpful for everyone in the family. For example, if you live in an urban or large suburban area, smog and other environmental pollutants can increase the body's production of harmful free radicals. Exposure to cigarette or cigar smoke can also increase free radical production in the body. Even the healthy habit of regular physical activity can increase the body's production of free radicals, and its need for antioxidants. Consider adding a high-quality children's multivitamin to your child's daily routine to boost their intake of beta-carotene, vitamin C, vitamin E and other nutrients that deliver essential antioxidant protection.

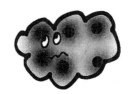

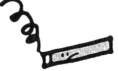

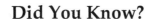

Did You Know?

Kids have a natural preference for how they learn whether it's by seeing, hearing or doing. Tap into your child's preferred method, and learning will seem almost effortless.

Tapping into Memory-Enhancing Sleep

You can maximize the power of a stress-free brain with memory-enhancing sleep. Yes, memory-enhancing. Sleep and memory experts have long known that getting enough zzz's after a day filled with learning is essential for converting those new skills into lasting memories. Researchers call this process memory consolidation. But, sleep also appears to help restore previous lost memories and produce additional memories all without the need for further practice. What's more, memory enhancement appears to occur largely while we're asleep.

Just what kind of sleep triggers all these memory benefits? It's REM sleep, the so-called deep sleep characterized by rapid eye movements. Throughout the night, we tend to alternate between memory-boosting REM sleep and non-REM sleep every 90 minutes or so. That means, with a good night's sleep, your child's brain has the opportunity to actively process the day's events, strengthen memory and possibly gain new insights about learned activities.

So, no matter what's on your child's daily To-Do list—studying for a spelling test, preparing for a piano recital or perfecting the latest skateboard move—make sure a day of learning is followed by a full night of restorative sleep. Read on for five essential steps to help promote memory-enhancing REM sleep.

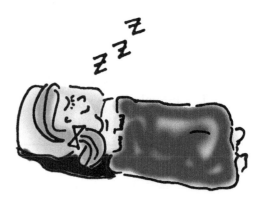

5 Steps to Memory-Enhancing Sleep

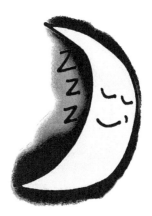

1 **Get enough hours of sleep each night.** The amount of sleep your child needs depends on their age. Typically, preschool children should sleep between 10 and 12 hours, while older children and teens need at least nine hours to feel fully refreshed and well rested.

2 **Keep bedtime the same time.** Going to bed at the same time will shape a sleep-promoting schedule.

3 **Keep the bedroom cool, dark and quiet.** Make sure your child's bedroom has the basics for a comfortable night's sleep: cool temperature, dark room and minimal noise.

4 **Limit fluids after dinner.** This will help reduce the need to wake up for those midnight trips to the bathroom. Should nature call, consider using a night-light to help guide the way.

5 **Avoid caffeine-containing drinks.** It's best for kids to avoid caffeine-containing foods and beverages because the stimulating effects of caffeine can last for several hours after that last sip is consumed. Its effect is so powerful, caffeine is the main ingredient in a wide variety of over-the-counter drugs designed to fight fatigue. So, when it comes to helping your little one drift off into sound slumber, the less caffeine consumed, especially after 3 p.m., the better.

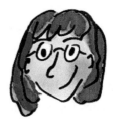

Did You Know?

Sleep experts at the National Sleep Foundation agree that watching television too close to bedtime not only makes it difficult for kids to fall asleep, but can also rob them of the much needed total hours of sleep. Aim to turn off the television—and all other electronics for that matter—at least one to two hours before bedtime. For more tips on promoting a happy slumber for kids and adults alike, visit www.sleepfoundation.org.

This Month's Smart Goal

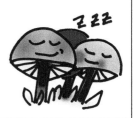

I will enforce a regular bedtime hour to help my child get enough memory-enhancing REM sleep at least five times per week.

This Month's Extra Credit

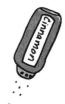

I will sprinkle an antioxidant-rich spice on my child's food each day or include a daily serving of a "Star Power" food (see list on page 83).

To monitor your daily progress toward your goals, use the **My Smart Tracker** forms in Chapter 14: Go for the Goal!

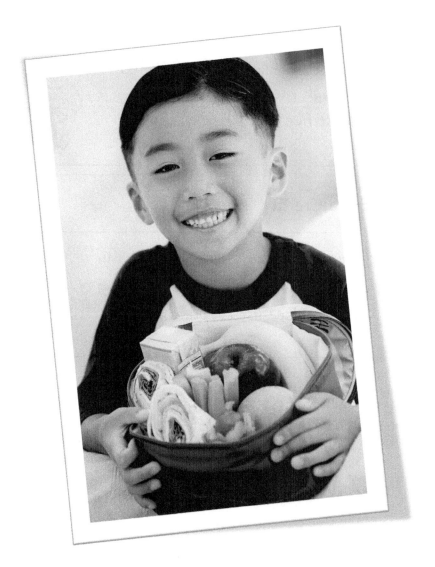

Listen to the mustn'ts, child. Listen to the don'ts.
Listen to the shouldn'ts, the impossibles, the won'ts.
Listen to the never haves, then listen close to me ...
Anything can happen, child. Anything can be.
                                        – *Shel Silverstein*

Chapter 6

January – Pack a Power Lunch

Can you believe it? The school year is almost half over. As time marches on, your beginning-of-the-year exuberance about packing your child's school lunch may be fizzling out. If you need a little inspiration to jazz up your menus, this chapter is for you. You'll learn new ways to revitalize the mid-day meal with both brain-building nutrition and kid-friendly flavor—to satisfy both you and your child.

While a healthy breakfast gets your kid's engine revving for their morning classes, lunch provides critical fuel for the home stretch. In fact, packing a power lunch is essential for your child to maintain focus and attention during those afternoon classes. It's easier than you may think when you focus on the nutrition essentials for energy, alertness and memory. Read on to learn more.

Carbs for Energy

Foods rich in carbohydrates provide the fuel to keep your child active throughout the school day. There are two types of carbohydrates: simple and complex.

Simple Carbohydrates

Simple carbohydrates provide quick energy.
Chemically speaking, simple carbohydrates are made up of
only one or two building blocks of sugar. Because of their
simple structure, it doesn't take long for them to break
down, be absorbed and used for energy in your child's body. This is the reason they
are often referred to as "quick energy." Examples include sucrose (white table sugar),
fructose (fruit sugar) and lactose (milk sugar). Each of these simple sugars end with
the letters "ose," which simply means sugar.

Complex Carbohydrates

Complex carbohydrates are made up of chains of
simple sugars and provide long-sustaining energy.
Before complex carbohydrates can be absorbed and
utilized in your child's body, they must first be
broken down.

It all starts with amylase, a digestive enzyme that helps slowly break down the
carbohydrate—releasing one sugar molecule at a time. Once a sugar molecule is
broken off, it can be absorbed and used by the body for energy. Because this process
takes time, it results in the sustained increase in energy that complex carbohydrates
provide. Foods rich in complex carbohydrates include bread, starchy vegetables,
cereals and other grain products.

Your Best Bets

The best carbohydrates are those that come from
unrefined sources. Think fruits and vegetables in terms of
simple carbohydrates. Think beans, legumes and
100% whole grains in terms of complex carbohydrates.
These choices are richer in vitamins, minerals, fiber and
phytonutrients.

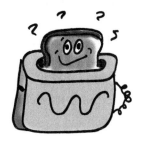

Think of a Pearl

You can help your child understand the concept of simple and complex carbohydrates by using a pearl analogy.

Ask your child to think of a pearl. It's like the simple carbohydrates (simple sugars) found in sodas, sweets, fruits, milk and similar foods. Let your child know that this type of carbohydrate melts in the mouth and is quickly absorbed by the body. It provides a short burst of energy, but can be followed by fatigue.

Now, ask your child to imagine a strand of pearls. It's like a complex carbohydrate. When you string simple sugars together—like a strand of pearls—they become a complex carbohydrate. In order for the body to use complex carbohydrates for energy, it must break off one simple sugar at a time. It's like taking one pearl at a time off a pearl necklace. Since this is a slow process, energy is released slowly over time to deliver long-lasting energy. This is one of the key reasons why complex carbohydrates are the preferred fuel for your child's body.

Quality Counts

You can take this analogy one step further. Just as fake pearls are lower quality than their genuine counterparts, simple sugars from refined sources are lower quality, providing empty calories and little, if any, nutritional value. By contrast, the unrefined simple sugars found in fruits and vegetables are like a genuine pearl—high quality nutrition bundled with vitamins, minerals and phytonutrients.

Similarly, unrefined complex carbohydrates found in whole grains are like a genuine pearl necklace—high quality and bundled with vitamins, minerals and dietary fiber. And, just like a genuine pearl necklace looks better over time, unrefined carbohydrates—whether simple or complex—are better for the body over time.

Protein to Stay Alert

Protein is important for strong muscles, but did you know that it also helps keep your child alert? This is especially important in the mid-afternoon when kids tend to start dragging, and their attention begins to wander.

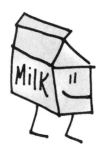

Protein-rich Brain Foods

- Milk, yogurt, cheese, egg whites
- Lean meat, poultry, fish, tofu
- Dried peas and beans, lentils, other legumes
- Nuts, seeds

Limit Saturated Fats for Memory

Your child needs an adequate intake of healthy fats, but too much fat, especially saturated fats, may impair the ability to pay attention, according to emerging laboratory research. Saturated fats include butter, lard, hydrogenated oils and other fats that remain solid at room temperature.

In a study published in the scientific journal *Neurobiology of Aging*, Dr. Carol Greenwood and her colleagues at the University of Toronto reported that the chronic ingestion of a high-fat, high-saturated fat diet actually impaired cognitive performance in laboratory rats. The researchers believe that a high-fat diet interferes with the body's ability to properly use blood sugar. These findings are preliminary, but there is plenty to suggest the same may be true for people.

It's Your Pick!

If your child continually brings home a lunch pail that's barely touched, it's time to join forces. Picky eaters tend to eat more when they do the picking.

If your child is a picky eater, enlist his or her help. Invite your child to pick one food in the four main food groups—a vegetable, a fruit, a protein-rich food and a food rich in complex carbohydrates.

Don't forget to include a healthy "drink pick" as well as a special treat or a "fun pick." Your child will feel valued that you are listening, and you'll be pleased to know that nourishing foods are fueling the day's learning. Read on to learn more about each "pick" list.

> **Parent Pearl**
>
> **Use your imagination.** My daughter has come up with all sorts of combinations for her lunch pail from apple slices with cinnamon to her own stackable creations with whole wheat crackers, cheese and luncheon meat. I have learned that my fussy eater will eat much more when she feels in charge of lunch.

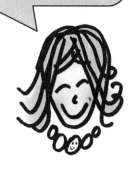

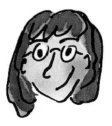

Did You Know?

If the newest sugar-laden cereal, high-fat snack or calorie-packed treat is just too enticing for your kids, establish a "dessert only" rule. Serve it up as an occasional dessert treat. The kids won't feel deprived, and you'll be helping keep their sugar intake to a minimum.

Vegetable Picks (phytonutrient-rich)

- Broccoli, cauliflower, jicama or other veggies cut into bite-size pieces
- Baby carrots (pre-washed and ready-to-go to save time during the early morning rush) or shredded carrot in a tuna sandwich
- Cherry tomatoes (rich in heart-healthy lycopene, and a beautiful and tasty combination when mixed with blueberries)
- Cucumbers
- Seaweed (can be found in convenient single-serving portions)
- Soybeans (often found in the frozen section; toss into a plastic bag in the morning to perfectly defrost for snack or lunchtime)
- Snap beans (kids love these little treasures)
- Sweet bell pepper (cut in strips)
- And many, many more!

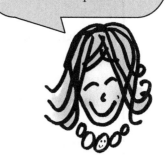

Parent Pearl

Check out your local kitchen tool supply shop. There are all sorts of utensils available to turn the shape of plain old carrot and celery sticks into fancy stars or other fun shapes.

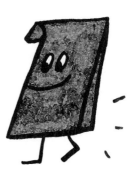

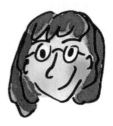

Did You Know?

Kids prefer vegetables cut into smaller pieces because they look less intimidating. You can tap into this natural preference to entice your child to eat more, even at school lunches. Pack colorful, bite-sized vegetables with a small container of hummus or other low-fat dip, and your child is sure to start munching more.

Fruit Picks (phytonutrient-rich)

- Apple
- Apple sauce (no sugar added)
- Banana
- Blueberries and other berries
- Cherries
- Fruit cocktail (packed in natural juices)
- Grapes
- Mandarin orange
- Melon chunks (you name it— cantaloupe, honeydew, watermelon, cassava)
- Orange slices
- Peach slices
- Pear
- Pineapple slices
- Plums
- Raisins
- Strawberries
- Tangerine
- And many, many more!

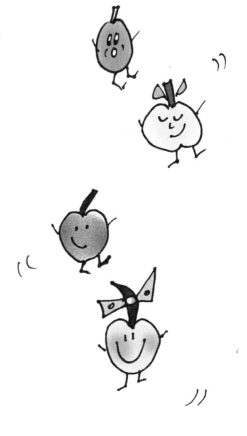

Note: It's best to avoid fruit roll ups since these choices stick to teeth and increase the risk of tooth decay and cavities.

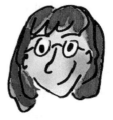

Did You Know?

You can help increase your child's fruit intake by choosing smaller pieces of fruit when shopping. Too often a big, delicious apple gets one bite and then is thrown away because the playground calls.

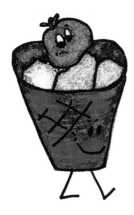

Protein Picks (aids alertness)

- Beans
- Beef jerky
- Cheese (low-fat string cheese or other low-fat choices)
- Chili
- Cottage cheese (non-fat or low-fat)
- Falafel
- Grilled chicken/chicken strips
- Hard-boiled egg
- Nuts, seeds
- Peanut butter (the natural-type) or other nut butters such as cashew, almond or soy (combine with 100% fruit spread, sliced apple or banana, or raisins)
- Stew
- Trail mix (buy a big bag and place small portions into snack-size plastic bags)
- Tuna or salmon (rich in omega-3 fats)
- Turkey, chicken, ham or other low-fat or non-fat luncheon meat
- Yogurt (non-fat or low-fat; plain or flavored)

Parent Pearl

Make enough for leftovers. When preparing dinners, I make extra pasta or other main dishes. The leftovers are a great (and easy) addition to my child's packed lunch for the next day.

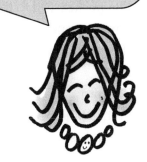

Carbohydrate Picks (for sustained energy)

- Bagel
- Cereal (consider a handful of cereal in a bag)
- Crackers
- English muffin
- Granola bar (choose whole grain bars portioned for kids)
- Muffins (make your own with your child's favorites—sunflower seeds, walnuts, raisins, cranberries, flax, shredded carrots or apple sauce—store in the freezer, pack one during the morning lunch prep, and it will be perfectly thawed by lunch)
- Pasta such as macaroni, noodles, spaghetti and others
- Pita chips
- Pita pockets (fill to the brim with sprouts, cucumbers, tomatoes and other fresh vegetables. Include a slice of cheese and/or luncheon meat for a protein boost.)

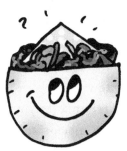

- Pizza
- Popcorn
- Pretzel (and peanut butter dip)
- Rice cakes
- Sandwich
- Soup (fill a thermos full of your child's favorite veggie or bean soup—a hit on a cold, blustery day)
- Starchy vegetables such as potato, corn, beans and peas
- Whole grain bread and rolls (pair up with hummus or low-fat cheese)
- Whole wheat tortillas (make a wrap with beans, cheese, turkey or chicken and top with tomato, avocado, pepper or cheese, or make a quesadilla with low-fat cheese)

Drink Picks (hydration boosters)

- Fruit juice such as apple, aronia, blueberry, boysenberry and pomegranate (consider adding a little sparkling water—approximately 3 parts juice to one part water—and make your own better-for-you soda)
- Fruit smoothie in a thermos
- Lemonade
- Milk (low-fat or non-fat; white or flavored)
- Rice milk
- Soy milk
- Vegetable juice
- Water

Note: Avoid fruit drinks, which are nothing more than refined sugar. Limit fruit juice to no more than ½ to ¾ cup per day for children, 1 to 6 years old, and no more than 1 to 1½ cups daily for older kids.

Parent Pearl

Consider buying a thermos or two. Over the course of the school year, this one purchase has saved me a bundle. With two, I always have one ready to use if the other is in the dishwasher. It also saves time during our hectic school mornings.

Fun Picks (for a special treat)

Lunch is always so much sweeter when you open your lunch box to find a fun surprise. Consider writing a love note, joke, riddle, drawing or brainteaser on your child's napkin. Sports clips and comics are also great to include to encourage reading. What's more, your child's friends are likely to look forward to finding out what's inside the "fun" lunch pail.

Consider planning ahead and collecting a stash of fun riddles and jokes from books or online sources. You'll avoid feeling stressed for time, and it will be a cinch to regularly include one in your child's lunch pail for a fun little extra to enjoy at lunch time.

Parent Pearl

Make fun sandwich shapes with cookie cutters. I reach for my heart-shaped cookie cutter to shape my kids' sandwiches into a special surprise just to say, "I love you!"

This Month's Smart Goal

I will have my child help out with the planning and making of school lunches at least once a week.

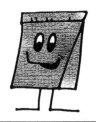

This Month's Extra Credit

I will include a joke, riddle, brainteaser or other fun pick in my child's lunch box at least twice a week.

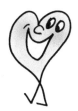

To monitor your daily progress toward your goals, use the **My Smart Tracker** forms in Chapter 14: Go for the Goal!

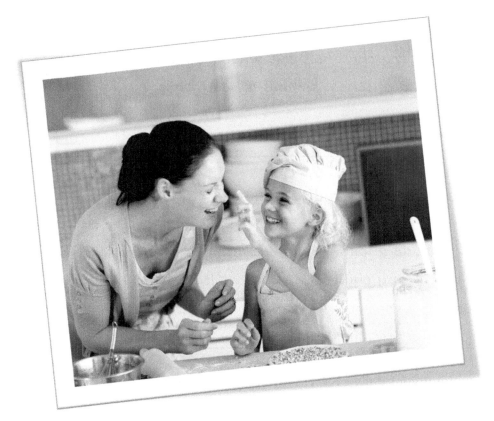

Find something you're passionate about
and keep tremendously interested in it.
– Julia Child

Chapter 7

February – Kids in the Kitchen

Exposing your child to an enriching environment is one of the best ways to sharpen their mind. What fits the bill better than cooking in the kitchen? Cracking an egg can challenge dexterity while providing an opportune time to talk to your child about choline, the brain-building nutrient found in eggs. You can challenge math skills by asking your child to double the ingredients in a favorite cookie recipe. Let your child convert kitchen equivalents—3 teaspoons per tablespoon, 2 cups per pint and 16 ounces per pound. You can even ask your child to read a recipe aloud to build confidence in public speaking. Even the very littlest helper can join in on the kitchen fun. Give them pots, pans and spoons to pretend to measure out an ingredient or even bang out a happy kitchen tune. The opportunities are endless, and your time is well spent. After all, taking the time to teach children to cook not only helps build a skill for life, but it also gives them an opportunity to share what's really going on in their lives.

The checklists that follow will help you choose age-appropriate tasks that are sure to inspire your child's inner chef—one step at a time!

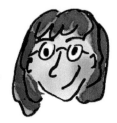

Did You Know?

Cooking with your child is the perfect time to practice volumes. Use measuring cups and spoons, clearly marked, to help reinforce the equivalent measures:

3 teaspoons = 1 tablespoon
16 tablespoons = 1 cup
2 cups = 1 pint
2 pints = 1 quart
4 quarts = 1 gallon

Inspiring Your Child's Inner Chef
(Kindergarten to 3rd Grade)

Check (☑) the box for each task your child has already tried. Place an X (☒) in the box for each new task to try.

- ❑ Adding ingredients
- ❑ Dropping cookie dough on trays
- ❑ Frosting cupcakes
- ❑ Husking corn (tiny fingers are perfectly suited to remove the hairs from the cob)
- ❑ Kneading dough
- ❑ Peeling hard boiled eggs
- ❑ Pouring cold liquids
- ❑ Reading recipes out loud
- ❑ Rolling dough
- ❑ Shelling peas
- ❑ Spreading peanut butter or jelly on bread
- ❑ Stirring
- ❑ Tearing lettuce into pieces for a salad
- ❑ Washing fruits and veggies

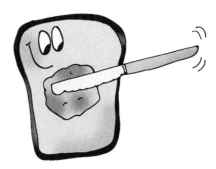

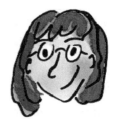

Did You Know?

You can help keep everyone safe in the kitchen while you enjoy cooking by following a few simple rules:

1. Use aprons.
2. Avoid wearing baggy clothes, including shirts with long, loose sleeves.
3. Put long hair back in a ponytail.
4. For older children, establish an age-appropriate "no touch" rule for knives and other sharp utensils; for younger children, keep sharp utensils away and out of sight.
5. At the stove, keep the handles of pots and pans away from the edge, turning them inward toward the stove.
6. Cook hot foods on the back burners, if possible.
7. Always supervise when fire or knives are in use.
8. Turn off the stove when finished.

Inspiring Your Child's Inner Chef
(4th Grade to 6th Grade)

Check (☑) the box for each task your child has already tried. Place an X (☒) in the box for each new task to try.

- ❑ Cracking eggs; separating whites from yolks
- ❑ Cutting fruits and veggies
- ❑ Filling muffin tins
- ❑ Helping to plan meals
- ❑ Helping to modify a recipe
- ❑ Measuring and mixing ingredients
- ❑ Peeling vegetables
- ❑ Reading food labels
- ❑ Reading recipes out loud
- ❑ Setting the table
- ❑ Using the can opener, blender and microwave
- ❑ Using a whisk
- ❑ Washing dishes

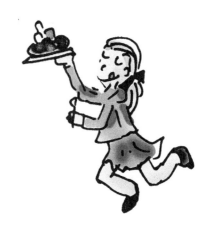

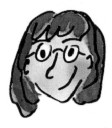

Did You Know?

Smell is one of our most powerful senses and can trigger memories from decades ago. Think of how the sweet smell of fresh citrus can bring you back to your childhood romps through an orange grove. You can help your child form these same feel-good memories by using aromatic foods in your recipes—cookies made with pure vanilla, bread baked with fresh rosemary or lemonade juiced from whole lemons.

10 Simple Tips for Cooking Success

Make your time in the kitchen a smashing
success with a few easy-to-use tips. Read on to
learn more.

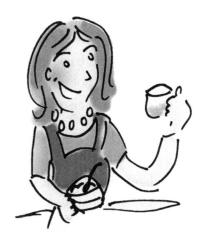

1 **Loosen up.** The key to any successful cooking
adventure is to choose a time when you're
both relaxed. An ideal time would be a lazy
weekend morning or a weekday afternoon after
homework is finished. Block off your calendar,
turn up the music and have fun!

2 **Ask your child to read the recipe to you.** This will help ensure that each step is
understood before beginning and that no emergency runs to the grocery store
are in order.

3 **Safety at all times.** Set ground rules to emphasize the importance of safety.
Teach kindergartners to avoid touching hot stovetops and pans, whirring
blenders and sharp knife blades. Discuss what's OK to touch and what's off limits.
Remind older children as well. Safety will go a long way toward making the most of
your special kitchen time.

4 **Scrub-a-dub-dub.** Before working with food, make sure all little hands are
properly washed. Here's how: Wet hands under
warm water, lather up with soap, wash for at least
30 seconds and rinse. To keep track of time, sing the
alphabet song—it's just about the right amount of time to
ensure a thorough cleaning. If a recipe calls for meat, fish
or poultry, be sure to also wash hands immediately after
handling.

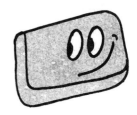

5 Clean as you go. An uncluttered kitchen makes for a more enjoyable experience. Teach your youngster to put containers of food back as you use them and to clean up as you go. This will not only keep your space free of clutter as you cook, but will also make cleaning up at the end a breeze.

6 Fresh is best. Use the freshest ingredients possible. We can't stress this enough. The wonderful aromas and flavors lend an irresistible joy to handling ingredients that are at their seasonal peak—a tomato plucked from the vine, a fresh sprig of dill or a pineapple bursting with juice.

7 Cut the fat and sugar; boost the fiber. Most likely, your treasured recipes rely on fat or sugar for a flavorful impact. Yet, it may only take a slight adjustment to make them healthier without affecting the flavors that your family loves. For recipe makeover inspiration, review our **Recipe Makeover Tips & Tricks** in Chapter 15: Tables, Tips & More.

8 Tools of the trade. Having the proper kitchen tools on hand can make the difference between enjoying your time in the kitchen and dreading it. Check out our **Choosing Kitchen Utensils & Tools** in Chapter 15: Tables, Tips & More to help you set up your winning kitchen.

9 Be prepared. Don't leave your cupboards bare. Be ready for whipping up a quick meal before your child's hunger strikes or if unexpected guests drop by. Need inspiration to get started? Check out our **Stocking Your Fridge, Freezer & Pantry** in Chapter 15: Tables, Tips & More.

10 **Praise.** There will be spills and messes as you go. It's just part of the learning process. Take it in stride and enjoy your precious time together. When you catch your child doing something right, be ready with lots of praise—the more specific the better. It will help build self-esteem and increase the odds that your child will want to spend more time in the kitchen. Who knows, you might have a future master chef in the making!

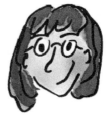

Did You Know?

The Centers for Disease Control and Prevention (CDC) provides an online tool to simplify recipe modification. Enter the main ingredients in your recipe and follow the prompts to retrieve healthful alternatives.

Learn more at www.fruitsandveggiesmatter.gov. Click "Interactive Tools" and then "Recipe Remix."

Vocabulary-Building Cooking

Build vocabulary while you cook. Here's how: Grab an ingredient, and ask your child to describe it using one-word adjectives. Choose words using all the senses—sight, smell, touch, taste and hearing. Check out the list below for inspiration.

acidic   appealing   appetizing   aromatic   astringent   bitter

bland   brittle   bumpy   chewy   chilly   cold   crisp

crystals   crunchy   crusty   delicious   delectable   delightful

doughy   dry   flavorsome   flat   fluid   frosty   frozen

glossy   gooey   gummy   hard   healthy   heavy   hot   icy

juicy   leathery   light   luscious   lukewarm   liquid   long

melting   mild   moist   mouth-watering   mushy   peppery

plump   pungent   rough   round   salty   scrumptious   sharp

shiny   slick   slushy   smoky   smooth   soggy   soft   sour

spicy   spotted   sticky   stringy   strong   succulent   sugary

sweet   syrupy   tangy   tart   tasteless   tasty   tender

tough   tepid   vinegary   viscous   warm   wet   weak

wilted   yucky   yummy   zesty

Fill Your Plate for Performance

Teach your child how to fill their plate with foods that give them energy and enhance performance. Here's how:

1 Ask your child to look at their plate and draw an imaginary line down the middle.

2 Explain that one half of the plate is devoted to non-starchy veggies such as spinach, tomatoes, carrots, zucchini and beets, just to name a few.

3 Once filled, ask your child to draw another imaginary line down the center of the empty half of the plate. Explain that one part is for protein-rich foods such as fish, chicken, meat or tofu, and the other part is for grains or starchy foods.

4 Top the meal off with a glass of low-fat or non-fat milk and a piece of fruit, and your child is ready to conquer his or her world!

You can even add some fun to the learning process with our **Rate Your Plate** game on page 119.

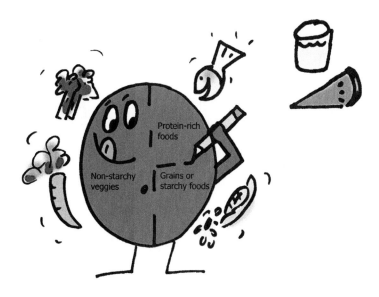

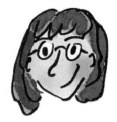

Did You Know?

You can teach your child to set the table like a pro in six easy steps. Here's how:

1. Place the plate in the center.
2. To the left, add the forks. If a salad fork is needed, place it to the far left since it's used first.
3. To the right, place the knife (blade toward the plate) and the spoon to the far right.
4. Slide the plate to one inch from the edge of table.
5. Add a napkin under the fork(s) or on the plate.
6. Finish by adding a cup to the upper right of the setting.

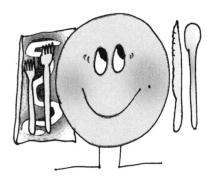

Rate Your Plate Game

Rate Your Plate is a fun game to help your child learn about healthy food choices and proper serving sizes. Get the entire family involved. The rules are simple. Check out the five healthy choices below. Each one earns one or more points. Whoever scores the most points is the mealtime winner!

1 point for <u>each</u> fruit or vegetable

1 point for <u>each</u> fruit or vegetable of a different color

1 point for a milk, cheese or other dairy product

1 point for a whole grain food

1 point for a protein-rich food

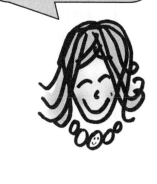

Parent Pearl

I love my pannini press. It's so easy to make an extra tasty sandwich, while at the same time packing in plenty of veggies. The flavors blend so well, and the kids often ask for more!

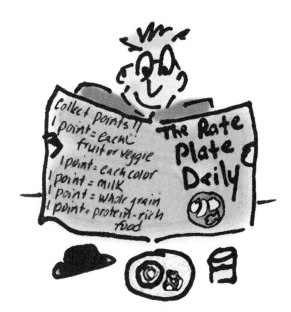

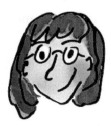

Did You Know?

You're just a click away from a great online resource for parents where you'll find tips on smart shopping, healthy cooking and eating right. It's called Kids Eat Right.

The nutrition experts at the Academy of Nutrition and Dietetics help sponsor this website, making it a must-have resource for reliable information. For more information, visit www.eatright.org/kids.

The Apple Doesn't Fall Far from the Tree

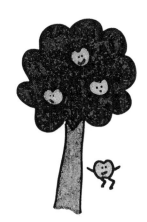

If you have a picky eater, take a look at yourself—picky eating may be a genetic trait. Dr. Lucy Cooke of University College London and her research team examined the eating habits of over 5,000 pairs of twins between the ages of 8 to 11 years and found that a child's aversion to trying new foods is mostly inherited. In fact, 78 percent of the aversion is considered genetic and a mere 22 percent is learned, according to a study published in the *American Journal of Clinical Nutrition*.

What's at the root of this food aversion? Earlier studies report that certain people have a genetic sensitivity to a bitter food compound called 6-n-propylthiouracil or PROP for short. The ability to taste PROP may play a role in a child's love-it or hate-it approach to broccoli, spinach, cabbage, Brussels sprouts and other bitter-tasting vegetables. What's more, kids who are PROP tasters are also reported to be more sensitive to sweet and pungent tastes as well as to the texture of fats.

In one study, researchers classified 65 preschool children as either PROP tasters (24 children) or PROP non-tasters (41 children). The children were invited to freely choose from among five vegetables including black olives, cucumbers, carrots, red pepper and raw broccoli. The result? As expected, the children who were PROP non-tasters consumed significantly more vegetables, especially the more bitter tasting vegetables, compared to the children with the super sensitive PROP-tasting palettes.

> **Parent Pearl**
>
> **Let the kids cook!** Once a month, I let the kids choose a meal to make. Their inspirations are incredible, plus it's priceless to see the smile on their face from a job well done!

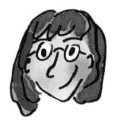

Did You Know?

Kids—like all of us—learn best by doing. When teaching your child a new skill in the kitchen, the wisdom of three applies:

1. First, let your child observe what you are doing.
2. Next, let your child do the same activity with your coaching; offering encouragement and guidance.
3. Finally, let your child try it solo.

Tips to Entice PROP Tasters

If your child is a PROP taster, he or she is sure to be super sensitive to bitter flavors and likely have some sensitivity to overly sweet and pungent flavors. To help entice his or her discriminating palette, consider trying one or more of the food preparation tips below:

- Stir-fry or otherwise lightly cook broccoli, cabbage and other bitter veggies to reduce the bitter bite.
- Grate, mince or puree carrots, zucchini, spinach and other veggies into pasta sauces, soups and quiches. The more you blend them, the less your child will recognize them.
- Lightly sweeten winter squash, carrots and other root vegetables with honey or brown sugar.
- Neutralize the taste of bitter salad greens with avocado or a little olive oil. Some bitter compounds dissolve when mixed with fats.
- Offer a dip or dressing with veggies.
- Sprinkle raw veggies with lemon juice or balsamic vinegar.
- Add a pinch of salt to veggies to help block the bitterness and enhance the sweetness.

Parent Pearl

To speed up meal prep when measuring spoons are missing, I simply use my thumb as a guide. From tip to first knuckle, your thumb is about one teaspoon. Simply multiply by three and you have a tablespoon.

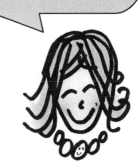

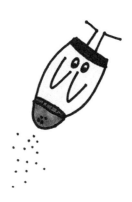

This Month's Smart Goal

I will have my child help create one complete meal for the family this month (grocery shopping, cooking and setting the table).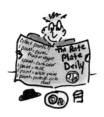

This Month's Extra Credit

I will play Rate Your Plate with my child at three meals per week (and earn at least 5 points per session).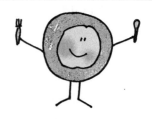

To monitor your daily progress toward your goals, use the **My Smart Tracker** forms in Chapter 14: Go for the Goal!

Part 4
Spring Fever

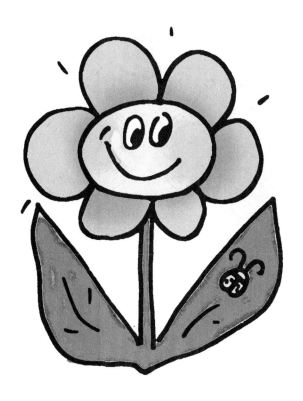

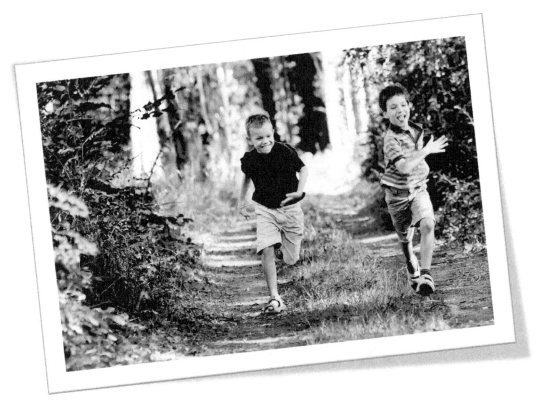

Genius is 1 percent inspiration
and 99 percent perspiration.
— Thomas Edison

Chapter 8

March – Fit Body, Fit Brain

If you think your child can fully exercise his or her brain just by studying, think again. Physical activity is also essential. It increases blood flow to the brain—bringing with it life-sustaining oxygen and the brain's preferred energy source, glucose.

Physical activity also triggers the production of chemicals, called nerve growth factors, which appear to extend the life of brain cells and increase their number and the connections between them. Exercise also activates brain cells to release serotonin and norepinephrine, two important biochemical messengers that help sustain attention and the ability to concentrate. The result: A brain that is more efficient and adaptive, which translates into better learning and performance for your child.

What Exercise Is Best?

While the brain accounts for only about 2 percent of your child's total body weight, it guzzles about 15 to 20 percent of the daily intake of oxygen and energy-producing calories. To deliver oxygen, calories and other nutrients to a hungry brain, your child relies on a healthy—and constant—flow of blood. What's the best way to get the heart pumping and blood flowing throughout the body and brain? You guessed it: Physical activity.

The good news is just about any physical activity will help increase blood flow to the brain. What's more, there's no shortage of enjoyable activities available to your child such as playing on the monkey bars, jumping rope or hopscotch, just to name a few. The trick is to let your child choose the most enjoyable activities—whether it's team-based or free play. Need inspiration to include more activity in your child's life? Check out our **Fitness from A to Z** list on the next page.

How Much Exercise?

There are 1,440 minutes in a day. The U.S. Department of Health & Human Services recommends that school-aged children spend at least 60 of those minutes engaged in some type of moderate to vigorous activity. To prevent obesity, experts recommend that most girls between the ages of 6 and 12 years maintain an activity level equal to about 12,000 steps per day, while boys need slightly more at 15,000 steps per day.

For some kids, this is an easy target, but for many, it can seem daunting. If your child sweats at the mere thought of 12,000 steps, be sure to take it slowly with small goals and make it extra fun. Remember, you're helping to build a healthy habit that your child will take into adulthood and likely pass on to their kids.

Approach exercise as play. As your child gets into better shape, the ability to move with greater coordination and agility is sure to bring a welcome surge in self-esteem and confidence, along with lots of smiles.

> ### Parent Pearl
>
> **Step it up.** My daughter loves her pedometer. She keeps track of her daily steps and is delighted when she breaks a new record. Being the competitive type, she also loves to challenge the rest of the family to a "step off," which helps keep everyone more active.

Fitness from A to Z

Check (☑) the box next to the activity that sounds like fun to your child. Choose one to try today.

❏ Aerobics

❏ Badminton

❏ Baseball

❏ Basketball

❏ Bowling

❏ Climbing

❏ Cycling

❏ Dance (Ballet)

❏ Dance (Jazz)

❏ Dance (Modern)

❏ Dance (Other)

❏ Dance (Tap)

❏ Dodge-Ball

❏ Duck, Duck, Goose

❏ Equestrian Events

❏ Four Square

❏ Frisbee

❏ Golf

❏ Gymnastics

❏ Handball

❏ Hiking

❏ Hockey

❏ Hopscotch

❏ Hula Hooping

❏ Ice Skating

❏ Inline Skating

❏ Jump Roping

❏ Kickball

❏ Kite Flying

❏ Lacrosse

❏ Martial Arts

❏ Monkey Bars

❏ Nature Walk

❏ Off-Road Biking

❏ Outdoor Activities

❏ Playing Catch

❏ Quarterback

❏ Red Light, Green Light

❏ Roller-skating

❏ Running

❏ Shuffleboard

❏ Skateboarding

❏ Skiing

❏ Snorkeling

❏ Snowboarding

❏ Soccer

❏ Softball

❏ Swimming

❏ Table Tennis

❏ Tag

❏ T-Ball

❏ Tennis

❏ Tetherball

❏ Ultimate Frisbee

❏ Volleyball

❏ Walking

❏ Xare (a racquetball game)

❏ YMCA activities

❏ Zoo Visit

❏ Zorbing (for the adventurous)

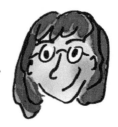

Did You Know?

Physical activity is directly linked to academic performance, according to a study published in the *Journal of Pediatrics*. William McCarthy, Ph.D., and colleagues at UCLA followed nearly 2,000 school-aged kids in grades 5, 7 and 9 to compare their aerobic fitness and body weight with their scores on California's standardized math, reading and language tests.

Dr. McCarthy's team found that those students who met California fitness standards (as measured by their time on a one-mile run/walk test) or who were at a healthy weight had higher average test scores than those students who did not—even after controlling for such factors as parent education and economic and social status.

Five Tips to Encourage Activity

1 **Walk to school.** Henry David Thoreau said it best: "An early-morning walk is a blessing for a whole day." If practical, walk your child to school. It has rewards well beyond physical activity—the giggles from seeing their face reflected in a puddle, the joy of discovering a new bug along the pathway or the delight of spotting a glorious sunflower smiling down from its high perch. And, you'll be making fond memories that will last a lifetime.

2 **Take charge.** Don't leave physical activity to the whims of others. Some schools or teachers may encourage enriching physical activities, but sadly, this is no longer the norm. Take charge by planning some of your family time around recreational activities—a hike, a bike ride, a friendly basketball or tennis challenge.

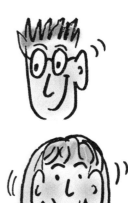

3 **Listen to your child.** Help your child choose an activity based on his or her activity temperament. If your child is a sports fan who thrives on competition and loves interacting with others, consider baseball, basketball, soccer, volleyball or other team sports. If your child prefers a more individual challenge, activities such as cross-country running, singles tennis, martial arts or gymnastics may be a better choice. If your child goes weak at the knees with the whole win/lose scenario, consider hiking, dancing, outdoor play and other activities that encourage a cooperative spirit.

4 **Limit TV to no more than two hours per day.** According to "Generation Play," a publication produced by the Stanford School of Medicine, 36 percent of young children up to 6 years of age have a TV in their bedroom. This figure soars to a whopping 68 percent for children between the ages of 8 and 18 years. If your child is begging for a TV for their room, we recommend that you stand firm and resist the temptation.

5 **Be a role model for good health.** If you want an active child, be active yourself. No amount of talking can ever replace the impact of watching a parent simply practice what they preach. It's the most powerful tool in your toolbox.

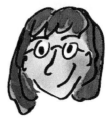

Did You Know?

Between television, computers, video games and phones, the amount of time kids spend in front of a screen—and inactive—is staggering. One recent study found that children and teens between the ages of 8 and 18 years spent almost 7 hours per day with personal use media such as television, DVDs, computers, radio and CDs. On average, the kids spent 4 hours a day watching TV, DVDs or videos.

Fueling Active Kids for Competition

Now that your child is active, your question may be, "What should I feed my child before a soccer game or other intense activity?" The types of foods that fuel your child's athletic performance are the same as those that fuel your child's brain for peak performance. The only difference may be in the timing.

In general, kids need to eat small meals throughout the day to optimize energy. When it comes to physical activity—especially intense training sessions, competitive games and other extremely vigorous activities—consider providing nourishment in the time intervals outlined below.

Three or four hours before a game or practice

Three to four hours before activity, have your child fill up on a carbohydrate-rich meal. For breakfast, consider oatmeal with slices of banana and a sprinkle of cinnamon, toast and a cup of steamy hot chocolate. For lunch, consider a turkey and veggie sandwich, milk and a piece of fruit. For dinner, consider a dish of marinara pasta with a sprinkle of cheese, a green salad, crisp apple slices and low-fat milk.

One hour before a game or practice

One hour before activity, give your child a snack. Consider a granola bar, four or five graham crackers, a half a bagel or a banana. It's also important for your child to be well hydrated. Make sure they drink at least 1½ cups (12 ounces) of water at this time.

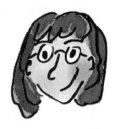

Did You Know?

If your child has more than one competitive athletic match during the same day, it's especially important to refuel between matches. A good rule of thumb is to eat 0.7 grams of carbohydrates per pound of body weight no later than 30 minutes after a match. For example, if your child weighs 75 pounds, a snack or meal with at least 53 grams of carbs is ideal. Here are a few kid-friendly options to consider:

Food	Carbohydrates
Apple (1 small)	15 grams
Orange (1 small)	15 grams
Banana (1 small)	15 grams
Berries (1 cup)	15 grams
Juice (½ cup)	15 grams
Sweet or white potato (3 ounces)	15 grams
Bread (1 slice)	15 grams
Bagel (¼ each or 1 ounce)	15 grams
Milk (1 cup)	12 grams
Yogurt (¾ cup)	12 grams
Granola or energy bar (1 each)	Varies (check label)
Sports drink (1 each)	Varies (check label)

During a game or practice

Keep the water flowing! Water is the best choice during and after a workout to rehydrate. Sports drinks are another popular option. They typically contain sodium and other electrolytes that can be lost in sweat during prolonged vigorous activity. But, the sugar-acid combo typically found in sports drinks can dramatically increase the risk of cavities and other dental issues. Be sure to keep water handy for a quick rinse. And, for less intense activity, water is best.

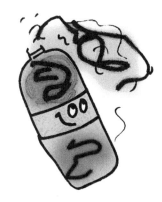

After a game or practice

After activity, rehydrate and refuel. Have your child drink plenty of water—about 2 cups (16 ounces) for every pound of body weight they have lost. In addition, have your child eat a carbohydrate-rich food within 30 minutes after the end of the workout. This is especially important for a competitive player who has more rounds of competition later the same day. It helps replenish the body's glycogen stores to fuel the next performance. Here, timing is key—don't wait too long—as the muscles are especially primed to store glycogen within 30 minutes of a vigorous bout of activity.

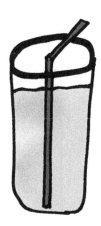

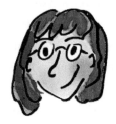

Did You Know?

Regular exercise makes kids smarter, according to a study published in *Research Quarterly for Exercise & Sports* involving over 90 overweight children between the ages of 7 and 11 years.

The researchers report that kids who participated in aerobic exercises for 40 minutes five times per week over a 15-week period scored significantly higher on a standardized test of cognitive processes compared to kids who did not participate.

Even better, the improvement in cognition was related to executive function—the ability to plan, initiate, self-monitor, self-control and carry out activity sequences that make up goal-directed behavior. This key cognitive function has the most dynamic growth during the elementary school years. So, it pays to play!

The Cost of Physical Inactivity

Regular physical activity plays a key role in helping your child maintain a healthy body weight, excel in school and build self-confidence. Conversely, physical inactivity and excess body weight have profound negative effects that sap the body, mind and spirit.

When it comes to excess body weight, the more overweight a child is, the more likely he or she will be absent from school, according to a study published in the journal *Obesity*. The researchers followed fourth to sixth grade students and found, on average, that underweight children were absent about 8 days, children at a healthy body weight were absent about 10 days, and overweight children were absent about 11 days. More research is needed to determine whether increased absences significantly affect an overweight student's performance, but it's certainly not a good trend to see.

What's a parent to do? First and foremost, be a role model and keep the lines of communication open. Next, continue to reinforce healthy habits with tools such as this book. Finally, reach out for additional resources. With childhood obesity at an all time high—about one out of every three kids in the United States is now overweight—experts are redoubling their efforts to address this serious public health concern. The result is more resources and tools will be developed to help families, schools and communities tackle childhood obesity.

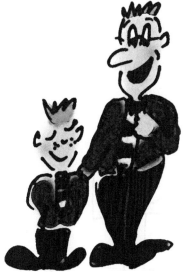

Is Your Child's Weight Healthy?

Your child's body mass index (BMI) estimates body fat using weight and height and is a good predicator of overall health. To determine your child's BMI, use an online tool such as the Child and Teen BMI Calculator at the Centers for Disease Control and Prevention's website (http://apps.nccd.cdc.gov/dnpabmi/) or calculate it from scratch using the steps below.

Step 1: Weigh your child and enter the amount in pounds below:

_____ (my child's weight in pounds)

Step 2: Measure your child's height in inches and enter the amount below:

_____ (my child's height in inches)

Step 3: Calculate your child's BMI using the following formula:

BMI = [weight ÷ (height)^2] x 703.

For example, a 50-pound child who is 48 inches tall has a BMI of 15.3:

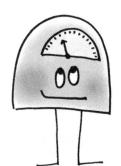

BMI = [weight ÷ (height)^2] x 703

BMI = [50 pounds ÷ (48 inches)^2] x 703

BMI = [50 pounds ÷ 2,304] x 703

BMI = 15.3

My child's BMI is:

BMI = [_____ pounds ÷ (_____ inches)^2] x 703

BMI = _____

Step 4: Select the BMI chart below for your child's gender (girl or boy). Find your child's age and determine which weight category the BMI falls into (i.e., underweight, healthy weight, overweight or obese).

Body Mass Index (BMI) Categories for Children				
Age	**Underweight**	**Healthy BMI**	**Overweight**	**Obese**
For Boys				
5 years	less than 13.9	13.9 up to 16.8	16.8 up to 17.8	17.8 or more
6 years	less than 13.8	13.8 up to 16.9	16.9 up to 18.1	18.1 or more
7 years	less than 13.7	13.7 up to 17.2	17.2 up to 18.8	18.8 or more
8 years	less than 13.7	13.7 up to 17.7	17.7 up to 19.6	19.6 or more
9 years	less than 13.9	13.9 up to 18.3	18.3 up to 20.6	20.6 or more
10 years	less than 14.1	14.1 up to 19.0	19.0 up to 21.6	21.6 or more
11 years	less than 14.4	14.4 up to 19.8	19.8 up to 22.7	22.7 or more
12 years	less than 14.8	14.8 up to 20.6	20.6 up to 23.7	23.7 or more
For Girls				
5 years	less than 13.5	13.5 up to 16.8	16.8 up to 18.2	18.2 or more
6 years	less than 13.4	13.4 up to 17.1	17.1 up to 18.8	18.8 or more
7 years	less than 13.4	13.4 up to 17.6	17.6 up to 19.6	19.6 or more
8 years	less than 13.5	13.5 up to 18.3	18.3 up to 20.6	20.6 or more
9 years	less than 13.7	13.7 up to 19.0	19.0 up to 21.7	21.7 or more
10 years	less than 14.0	14.0 up to 19.9	19.9 up to 22.9	22.9 or more
11 years	less than 14.4	14.4 up to 20.8	20.8 up to 24.0	24.0 or more
12 years	less than 14.8	14.8 up to 21.7	21.7 up to 25.2	25.2 or more
Source: Centers for Disease Control and Prevention (www.cdc.gov)				

How Many Calories Are Enough?

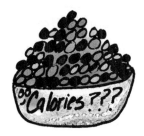

The number of calories your child needs to maintain a healthy body weight depends on a variety of factors such as activity level, gender, age, height and weight. Counting calories is generally not necessary, but knowing a ballpark number may help you plan a healthy diet. Remember to include a wide variety of nutritious foods from each food group in order to optimize brain and physical performance. You'll find details about your child's calorie and food needs in Chapter 15: Tables, Tips & More. Focus on two tables: **Recommended Daily Intake: Calories** and **Recommended Daily Intake: Food Groups.**

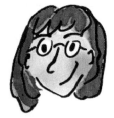

Did You Know?

You can serve age-appropriate portions by keeping an eye on portion distortion. When you serve larger portions, kids tend to take bigger bites and eat more. Some kids who have difficulty recognizing the feeling of fullness are specially prone to overeating when portions are large, which can lead to excess weight gain. Allowing children to choose their own portion size may help avoid gulping down large portions just because they're there.

Watch Out for Portion Distortion

Studies have found that our ability to judge the amount of food on our plate is affected by the size of the plate we use. A portion of food will appear smaller and more compact when it's served on a large, imposing plate. The same portion, however, will appear noticeably larger when served on a smaller plate. Why? Our brain makes a false assessment about the quantity of food. It's a visual illusion based on the principle of concentric circles.

In practical terms, the plate needs to be at least two-thirds full for your eye to feel satisfied. So what does this mean for you and your child? If your child is overweight, consider using a smaller plate so they don't feel deprived. Conversely, if you have a picky eater, consider using a larger plate so they don't feel overwhelmed with the amount of food on their plate.

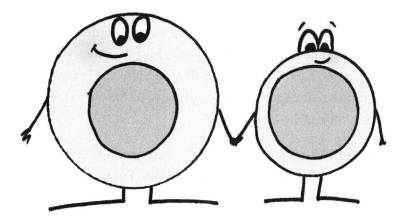

The principle of concentric circles. A portion of food will appear smaller and more compact when served on a large, imposing plate—a great choice to entice a picky eater. The same portion, however, will appear noticeably larger when served on a smaller plate— a great choice to help satisfy an overweight child.

5 Active Tips to Train the Brain for Greatness

1 **Tap into the e-revolution.** If you have a PlayStation® or other type of electronic wizard on your hands, consider purchasing games that get your child—and the rest of the family—jumping and sweating. Dance Dance Revolution®, a game available for PlayStation and other devices, is a great choice. In fact, it's part of the physical education curriculum in thousands of schools nationwide. The game is not only a great workout for the body, but also for the brain. You could even consider a family round of Dance, Dance Revolution or other active games to get the whole family rocking, hopping and rollicking.

2 **Watch the greats.** When you perform a task, your brain patterns are actually quite similar to when you're watching someone else perform the same task. So, not only does playing sports improve brain function, but according to research from the University of Chicago, watching sports can change the neural networks in the brain and improve brain function as well.

3 **If you can imagine it, you can be it.** Tap into the technique of visualization to help stimulate the brain. For example, if your child wants to learn basketball, encourage using the "mind's eye" to see the ball going into the hoop, hear the swoosh as it rolls around and experience the applause of the crowd. The more vivid the imagination, the stronger the effect.

4 **Use your head, don't hurt your brain.** Make sure your child has proper protection when participating in various activities. For example, ensure that helmets fit securely while cycling or playing football.

5 **Share a laugh.** Laughing stimulates the brain, so don't underestimate the value of the lighter side of life. Laugh a lot, and laugh often.

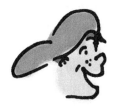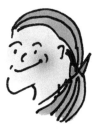

This Month's Smart Goal

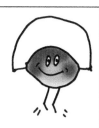

I will add 5 minutes of jumping, running or other fun activities until my child is active at least 60 minutes every day. (Take it one step at a time—listen to your child—and make sure it's fun!)

This Month's Extra Credit

I will help my child limit TV to no more than 2 hours per day.

To monitor your daily progress toward your goals, use the **My Smart Tracker** forms in Chapter 14: Go for the Goal!

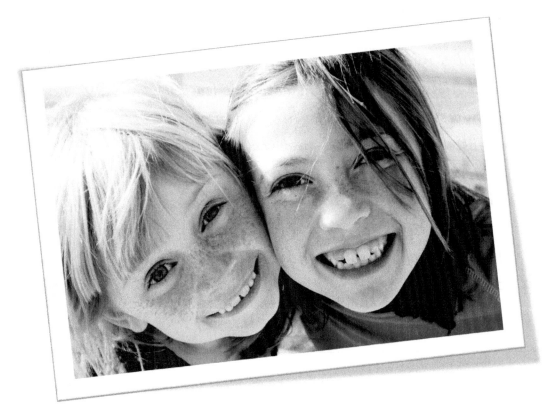

Nothing great was ever achieved without enthusiasm.
—Ralph Waldo Emerson

Chapter 9

April – Celebration beyond Cupcakes

With so many milestones to celebrate—birthdays, team victories, classroom achievements and more—your child is likely to be served plenty of cupcakes, cakes, cookies and similar sweets. In fact, no longer are these foods a small treat after enjoying more nutrient-dense foods, they now command center stage at most celebrations.

Trouble is, these foods are typically loaded with sugar, which packs a double whammy for your child: Empty calories and tooth decay. The good news is, with a little know-how, you can easily learn how to limit sugary foods and choose healthier options more often—without putting a damper on all the fun.

Limit Empty Calories

With childhood obesity at an all time high, it's more important than ever to focus on limiting your child's intake of sugary foods with empty calories. Not banish, just limit. In fact, nutrition experts report that every healthy diet can include a few empty calories.

Just how many calories add up to "a few"? Aim for no more than 10 percent of your child's daily calorie intake as empty calories—the fewer, the better. We call this the 10% Rule. In practical terms, this translates to no more than a few hundred calories each day—much less than one typical frosting-laden cupcake. Keeping these empty calories under control is a great way to help your child maintain a healthy body weight.

You'll find all the need-to-know details about the amount of total daily calories your child needs—and the 10% Rule to limit the intake of empty calories—in Chapter 15: Tables, Tips & More.

Smile Saving Strategy

When you use the 10% Rule to limit the intake of sugary foods, you'll not only help your child maintain a healthy body weight, but you'll help protect your child's teeth. Why? One of the main causes of tooth decay—in children and adults—is the total amount of time teeth are exposed to sugar. In the mouth, bacteria quickly transform sugar into acids that attack tooth enamel and cause tooth decay. Eating sugary foods throughout the day allows for plenty of acid-producing activity that can increase the risk of cavities. By contrast, the 10% Rule helps deny mouth bacteria the sugar it needs to do its dirty work. The result is likely to be fewer cavities and better dental checkups.

A Better Sweet for Your Sweetie

Some kids just love sweets. The trick is to find a healthier substitute that they love just as much. Read on for a few suggestions to inspire you to pass on the cake, candy and other sugary or high-fat foods and reach for nutrient-dense alternatives that pack a flavor punch.

Birthday cake

- ❑ Blueberry Mini Muffins*
- ❑ Brainy Banana Bread*
- ❑ Fresh fruit kabobs with fruit-flavored yogurt dip
- ❑ Fruity Yogurt Parfait*
- ❑ Going Coconuts for Pineapple Cake*
- ❑ Yummy Crumbly Crisp*

Chewy candy

- ❑ 100% xylitol or sorbitol-sweetened gum
- ❑ Chocolate bar (choose the mini ones for easier portion control)
- ❑ Crackers with old-fashioned peanut butter
- ❑ Dried fruit (apricots, raisins, mangoes, plums and others)
- ❑ Fresh fruit
- ❑ Fruit and nut bar
- ❑ Granola or trail mix
- ❑ Whole grain bar

Cookies

- ❑ Animal crackers
- ❑ Gingersnaps
- ❑ Graham crackers
- ❑ Unsweetened fruit-nut-seed bar
- ❑ Whole grain muffin or loaf

Donut, chips, churro

- ❑ Air-popped popcorn
- ❑ Bagel
- ❑ Nuts
- ❑ Seeds
- ❑ Soft pretzel
- ❑ Soynuts

Ice cream (premium)

- ❑ 100% fruit juice bar
- ❑ Frozen fudge bar
- ❑ Frozen grapes
- ❑ Lower fat ice cream
- ❑ Low-fat and non-fat frozen yogurt
- ❑ Unsweetened applesauce with non-fat cottage cheese

Milkshake, soda

- ❑ Banana Nutty Shake*
- ❑ Fruit spritzer
- ❑ Fruit smoothie
- ❑ Pudding
- ❑ Sweet Strawberry Nectar*

*See recipe at the end of this chapter.

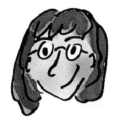

Did You Know?

Research supports the regular use of gum sweetened with xylitol or sorbitol to help prevent tooth decay. Unlike sugar, these sweeteners aren't used by mouth bacteria to churn out cavity-producing acids—a distinct advantage over gums sweetened with sugar. The act of chewing also helps stimulate a healthy flow of saliva, which protects tooth enamel. When your child asks for a sweet, reach for a gum sweetened with one of these smile savers. It's a win-win situation: Less sugar and a healthier smile.

Where Does Sugar Hide?

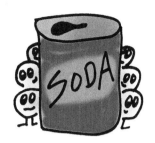

Sugar is naturally found in milk, fruit and other whole foods. But added sugar also hides in many processed and packaged foods. In fact, a typical child 4 years and older consumes more than 20 teaspoons of added sugar every day. That's over 320 extra calories—and it lurks in soda, ketchup and many other kid-friendly foods.

Food	Sugar
Soda, 12 ounces	10 teaspoons
Figs, 3 each	9½ teaspoons*
Fruit punch drink, 1 cup	7 teaspoons
Fruit juice, 6 ounces	6 teaspoons*
Coconut, sweetened, 2 ounces	5 teaspoons*
Gelatin, flavored, ½ cup	5 teaspoons
Chocolate, 1 ounce	4 teaspoons
Honey, 1 tablespoon	4 teaspoons
Yogurt, 1 cup	4 teaspoons*
Cereal, sweetened, 1 cup	3 teaspoons
Ice cream, ½ cup	3 teaspoons
Milk, 1 cup	3 teaspoons*
Donut, cake type, 1 each	1 teaspoon
Jam, 1 teaspoon	1 teaspoon
Ketchup, 1 tablespoon	1 teaspoon
Chewing gum, 1 stick	½ teaspoon
* Predominately naturally occurring sugar.	

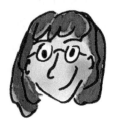

Did You Know?

You can help your child understand how much sugar is in packaged foods by teaching them to read labels. Here's how:

In the Nutrition Facts panel, find the number of grams of sugar per serving. For every 4 grams, your child is consuming the equivalent of 1 teaspoon of sugar.

You can also look in the Ingredient panel on the label to find the ingredients that contribute to the sugar content of the food. As a rule of thumb, foods with sugar listed among the top three ingredients tend to be high in sugar. Make sure these foods also have some fiber and protein. When sugar is accompanied by these two nutrients, it tends to have less of an effect on your child's blood sugar.

The Many Names of Sugar

The sugar in foods can masquerade under a wide variety of names. To spot the most common sugar-based ingredients found in packaged foods, simply look for the letters "ose" at the end of an ingredient's name such as dextrose, fructose, lactose, maltose, glucose, galactose and sucrose (white sugar), just to name a few.

Other common names for the sugar-based ingredients typically used to sweeten foods include barley malt syrup, brown rice syrup, brown sugar, corn syrup, high-fructose corn syrup, honey, lactitol, mannitol, maple syrup, molasses, raw sugar, sorbitol, sucanut, sugar alcohols (polyols), syrup and turbinado sugar.

Caution: Energy Drain Ahead

Foods high in sugar can provide a burst of quick energy, but the sharp energy drain that tends to follow can sap your child's ability to focus and concentrate. For staying power in the classroom, choose foods rich in complex carbohydrates, such as whole grains. These foods are absorbed more slowly, providing a steady source of fuel to keep active brains focused throughout the school day. What's more, these foods are likely to be more nutrient dense, delivering their slow carbs along with other nourishing vitamins, minerals and fiber.

Parent Pearl

Replace soda with a fruit spritzer. To satisfy my daughter's love for a a sweet, fizzy drink, I serve up a fruit spritzer. It's a healthier alternative to soda and so easy to make. I simply add a dash of carbonated water to her favorite fruit juice. For extra flair, I top it off with a slice of lemon or orange.

A caveat about soda

Neither diet nor regular sodas are a good choice for children, or adults for that matter. Regular sodas provide "empty calories" and contain nothing more than sugar (approximately 10 teaspoons per 12-ounce can), water, food coloring and flavor. Diet sodas do not contain calories, but they fail to provide any nutritional advantage. Better choices are water, non-fat and low-fat milk, and juice (in moderation).

The effect of excess sugar on learning

Diets loaded with sugar and fat, yet lacking in essential fatty acids, may lower the level of a critical bioactive compound in the brain involved in learning and memory. It's called brain-derived neurotropic factor (BDNF), and it's responsible for the development of new brain tissue and, therefore, for the formation of new memories.

Emerging research in laboratory rats reveals a direct link between the level of BDNF in the brain and the ability to learn spatial and memory tasks. What's more, when the laboratory rats were fed a diet high in sugar and fat, it only took two months to significantly reduce the level of BDNF in the brain and impact the animal's ability to perform spatial and memory tasks. More studies are needed to confirm a similar action in humans, but in the meantime, the findings add to the growing body of research that supports the brain benefits of avoiding excess sugar.

The Low Down on Sugar Substitutes

If you want to cut down on your child's sugar intake, you may be wondering about some of the sugar substitutes and sugar alternatives available in the marketplace.

Currently, the U.S. Food and Drug Administration (FDA) has approved six sugar substitutes for use in foods sold in the United States: acesulfame potassium, aspartame, neotame, saccharin, stevia and sucralose. The safety data for each of these sweeteners has been reviewed by national regulatory agencies, including the FDA, and by international health authorities, including the World Health Organization (WHO). The consensus is each sweetener is safe for use by all consumers, including children, pregnant women and people with diabetes.

Acesulfame potassium

Acesulfame potassium is a heat-stable sugar substitute that can be used in cooking and baking. It's used in combination with other sweeteners such as saccharin in carbonated low-calorie beverages and other products. It's also available as a tabletop sweetener. This sugar substitute is about 200 times sweeter than white sugar.

Aspartame

Aspartame is about 180 to 220 times sweeter than white sugar. It's not considered a "non-caloric" sweetener since it's broken down in the digestive tract into components that are absorbed and metabolized. However, because it's so sweet, just a small amount is needed to impart a big sweet taste. So, for all intents and purposes, the calories that it provides are negligible. A word of caution: Children with the rare genetic disorder called phenylketonuria or PKU must avoid this sweetener as they are unable to break it down.

Neotame

Neotame is one of the newest artificial sweeteners on the market and has a powerful sugary taste, approximately 7,000 to 13,000 times sweeter than white sugar.

Saccharin

Saccharin, the first artificial sweetener to market, is about 300 times sweeter than white sugar. It's found in many dietetic food and beverage products.

Stevia

Stevia comes from a plant and is about 250 to 300 times sweeter than white sugar.

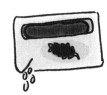

Sucralose

Sucralose is an artificial, non-caloric sweetener made from sugar. The body is unable to digest it, so it's excreted unchanged. It's about 600 times sweeter than white sugar.

Take home message

While all these sugar substitutes are FDA-approved options, we recommend that you reserve them for occasional use if you choose to use them at all.

As a general rule, we recommend that you choose whole foods whenever possible, rely on the natural sweetness of fruits and limit the intake of refined sweeteners.

Healthy Classroom Celebrations

With the rise in childhood obesity, more schools are encouraging parents to bring healthier foods for birthday and other celebrations during the school day. Here are a few options to consider for your child's next classroom celebration. Check with your child's teacher first, but we think the healthier options will be welcomed. Who knows, you just may start a trend.

Food items:

❑ Angel food cake, strawberries and whipped cream
❑ Carrot muffins (with just enough frosting for a smiley face)
❑ Fruit kabobs
❑ Pizza with 100% juice boxes
❑ Popcorn
❑ Pudding
❑ Snap peas or other veggies with a tasty dip
❑ Watermelon
❑ Yogurt parfait (see recipe on page 161)

Non-food items:

❑ A special book to read aloud and then donate to the class library
❑ Erasers
❑ Pencils
❑ Stickers
❑ Washable tattoos

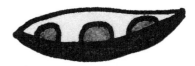

Tips to Reduce Refined Sugar

Check (☑) the box for each tip below you can include in your family's routine. Each tip helps cut the refined sugar in your child's diet. So, the more checks, the better.

❑ **Go au natural.** Buy fresh fruits or fruits packed in water or its own juice, rather than those packed in light or heavy syrup.

❑ **Buy fewer foods that are high in added sugar** such as prepared baked goods, candies, sweet desserts, soft drinks and fruit-flavored drinks.

❑ **Reduce the sugar in foods that you prepare at home.** Out of sight, out of mind. Start by reducing the sugar gradually until you've reduced it by one-third or more.

❑ **Add a pinch of salt.** It will enhance a food's natural sweetness.

❑ **Add less sugar.** Have your child add less sugar to cereal. It's easy to get used to using half as much.

❑ **Eat regular meals.** By offering meals and snacks throughout the day, you'll help curb your child's sweet tooth. Hunger is a sure-fire fiend that will tempt your child to eat a sugary snack.

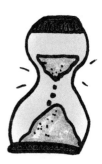

❑ **Buy breakfast cereals without added sugars.** Your child will consume less sugar even with a sprinkle of their own sugar on top. In fact, some breakfast cereals marketed to kids are more like a dessert with over 3 teaspoons of sugar per serving—and often kids don't stop at one bowl.

❑ **Read labels.** If sugar, in any of its many forms, is listed first on the ingredient list, use discretion or look for a healthier option.

❑ **Train taste buds to be accustomed to less.** By avoiding sugary foods for as little as one week, your child will be able to taste the natural sweetness in foods and be less tempted by sugary foods.

❑ **Keep within the empty-calorie limit and use wisely (see page 279).** These calories are limited, so choose foods that really count. For most kids, this means desserts. Don't waste these calories on sodas and sugary breakfast cereals.

❑ **Experiment with spices.** Cinnamon, cardamom, coriander, nutmeg, ginger, mace and other spices enhance the flavor of foods without adding sugar.

❑ **Serve sweet foods warm.** Heat enhances the perception of sweetness.

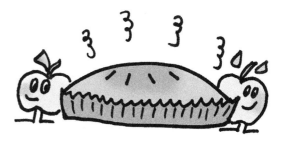

Banana Nutty Shake

This nutritious shake only needs four ingredients for a flavor burst that will have your child begging for more!

Ingredients

1 banana, frozen and broken into chunks
1 cup non-fat or low-fat milk
2 teaspoons honey
1 handful walnuts (about 6 halves)

Directions

1. In a blender, add banana, milk and honey.
2. Blend till smooth, about 45 seconds.
3. Add walnuts and blend for a few additional seconds.
4. Serve and enjoy!

Makes 2 servings (1 cup per serving)

164 **Calories** | 4g **Fat** | 26g **Carbs** | 6g **Protein**

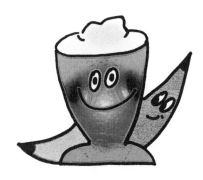

Blueberry Mini Muffins

This tasty breakfast addition or snack treat combines the antioxidant power of blueberries with hearty whole grain goodness and flaxseed, a natural source of omega-3 fats.

Ingredients

½ cup vanilla soymilk
½ cup apple juice concentrate
¼ cup canola oil
1 egg
1 cup whole wheat flour
1 cup oatmeal
¼ cup milled flaxseed

⅓ cup sugar
3 teaspoons baking powder
½ teaspoon salt
1 cup blueberries
¼ cup walnut, chopped

Directions

1. Preheat oven to 400 degrees.
2. Grease bottoms of 36 mini-muffin cups or line with paper baking cups.
3. In a bowl, beat soymilk, oil and egg. Stir in flour, oats, flaxseed, sugar, baking powder and salt until flour is moistened, but batter is lumpy. Fold in blueberries and nuts.
4. Divide batter evenly among muffin cups.
5. Bake for 15 minutes or until golden brown.
6. Remove immediately from pan to cool.
7. Serve and enjoy!

Freeze some for school lunches. Add a frozen muffin to the lunch box during morning prep time, and it will be perfectly thawed by lunch time.

Makes 36 servings (one muffin per serving)

55 **Calories** | 2g **Fat** | 8g **Carbs** | 1g **Protein**

Brainy Banana Bread

This tasty bread is sure to please even your most finicky critic.

Ingredients

½ cup sugar
¼ cup butter, softened
1 egg
2 bananas, mashed
¼ cup milk
¾ cup whole wheat flour
½ cup white flour

1 teaspoon vanilla
1 teaspoon cinnamon
4 tablespoons milled flaxseed
½ teaspoon baking soda
½ teaspoon salt
½ cup walnuts, chopped

Directions

1. Preheat oven to 350 degrees.

2. In a bowl, combine sugar and butter; mix well. Add egg, bananas, milk and flour; blend well.

3. Stir in remaining ingredients, except nuts, until just moistened.

4. Add nuts, but save a few for later.

5. Pour batter into a greased 8½x4½x2½-inch loaf pan.

6. Sprinkle top with remaining nuts. Bake for about 60 minutes or until a wooden toothpick inserted in the center comes out clean. Remove from pan to cool.

7. Cut into slices, serve and enjoy!

Makes 16 serving (1 slice per serving)

115 **Calories** | 4g **Fat** | 18g **Carbs** | 3g **Protein**

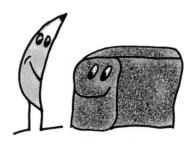

Fruity Yogurt Parfait

This colorful snack or dessert is a feast for the eyes and a rich source of protein and calcium.

Ingredients

6 ounces vanilla yogurt, or flavor of your choice

¼ cup granola

½ cup strawberries, or other favorite fruit, cut into slices

Directions

1. In a clear cup, alternate layers of yogurt, strawberries and granola.

2. Add a parasol for a colorful touch.

3. Serve and enjoy!

Makes 2 servings (¾ cup per serving)

160 **Calories** ǀ 3g **Fat** ǀ 28g **Carbs** ǀ 4g **Protein**

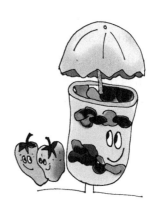

Going Coconuts for Pineapple Cake

When you have this tasty cake in the oven, don't be surprised if your little darling calls out, "Smells good, Mom!" You'll be pleased that the recipe calls for no added processed sugars.

Ingredients

Wet ingredients

½ cup chopped apricots, fresh or well-drained (about 6 medium)

¾ cup crushed pineapple, well-drained

½ cup apple juice concentrate

1 cup low-fat milk

2 eggs

¼ cup canola oil

1 teaspoon vanilla extract

Dry ingredients

2 cups whole wheat flour

⅓ cup unbleached white flour

1 teaspoon baking soda

3 teaspoons baking powder

2 teaspoons cinnamon

⅓ cup coconut, flaked

Optional (add with coconut)

8 apricots, dried, chopped

¼ cup walnuts, chopped

4 tablespoons milled flaxseed

Directions

1. Preheat oven to 350 degrees.

2. In a blender or food processor, add all wet ingredients and puree until smooth.

3. Place mixture in a large bowl and add the dry ingredients (except coconut). Beat well. Stir in coconut (and any optional ingredients).

4. Coat an 8x8-inch baking pan with vegetable spray and then pour in batter.

5. Bake for about 45 to 50 minutes or until an inserted toothpick comes out clean. Cool before cutting into slices.

6. Serve and enjoy!

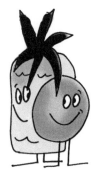

Makes 16 servings (1 slice per serving)

105 **Calories** | 6g **Fat** | 11g **Carbs** | 3g **Protein**

Sweet Strawberry Nectar

Talk about a winner. This fruit smoothie packs both flavor and nutrition, yet is oh-so-easy to whip up!

Ingredients

1 cup vanilla soymilk
5-6 strawberries, frozen
2 teaspoons whipped cream (optional)

Directions

1. In a blender, add soymilk and strawberries.
2. Blend until smooth, about 45 seconds.
3. Pour into cups, and if desired add a touch of whipped cream.
4. Serve and enjoy!

Consider buying a big bag of frozen strawberries, blueberries, blackberries or other berries, so you have plenty on hand.

Makes 2 servings (¾ cup per serving)

75 **Calories** | 1g **Fat** | 13g **Carbs** | 3g **Protein**

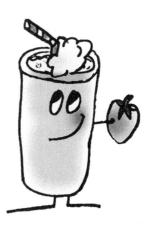

Yummy Crumbly Crisp

This delicious crisp is a snap to make.

Ingredients

⅓ cup butter, softened
½ cup brown sugar
1 teaspoon vanilla
½ cup flour
½ cup oats
¼ cup walnuts, chopped
6 cups sliced peaches (about 6 medium)*

Directions

1. Preheat oven to 375 degrees. Grease 11½x8x2-inch pan.
2. In a bowl, combine butter, brown sugar and vanilla. Add flour and oats. Mix well.
3. Stir in walnuts.
4. Place fruit in pan and sprinkle oat mixture over top.
5. Bake for about 30 minutes or until topping is golden brown.
6. Serve warm and enjoy! If desired, add a dab of fresh whipped cream.

Makes 9 servings

180 **Calories** | 8g **Fat** | 28g **Carbs** | 3g **Protein**

*Alternative: Use other fruits or a combination of fruits. Tasty combos include apples, nectarines and blueberries or pears and raspberries. Even slightly thawed frozen fruit works well. Use your imagination and have fun creating.

This Month's Smart Goal

I will help my child brainstorm a healthier substitute to one of his or her frequent junk food choices this month.

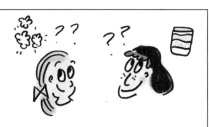

This Month's Extra Credit

I will help my child learn his or her recommended "empty calorie" limit.

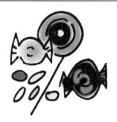

To monitor your daily progress toward your goals, use the **My Smart Tracker** forms in Chapter 14: Go for the Goal!

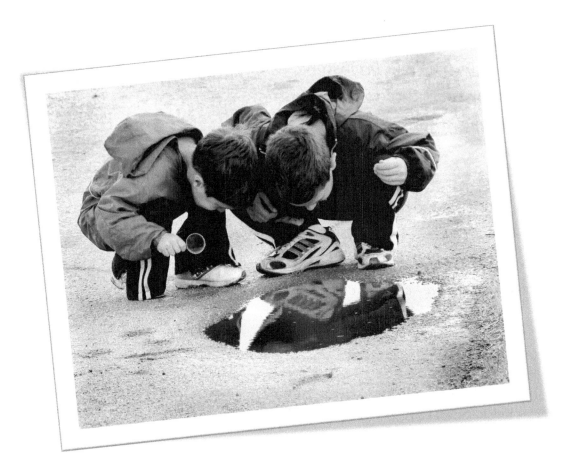

The belly rules the mind.
— Spanish proverb

Chapter 10

May – New Foods for Curious Minds

Introducing your child to new, healthy foods is a perfect way to stimulate an active mind while nourishing the brain. Trouble is, most kids turn their noses up at the mere mention of a food that's packed with brain-building nutrition—just because it's unfamiliar.

If your child is a picky eater, don't despair. Kids are actually hard-wired to avoid new foods, according to a study published in the *American Journal of Clinical Nutrition*. Researchers call this genetic trait food neophobia or a fear of new foods. They believe the trait may have developed to help us avoid unfamiliar foods that could be poisonous. For cavemen who relied on hunting and gathering for food, this initial aversion to unfamiliar foods was a good thing.

Today, however, our foraging is typically limited to trips to the local supermarket or farmer's market where foods are generally safe. So, in today's world, food neophobia actually works against us because it can limit the variety of nutrient-dense foods we eat, including fruits and vegetables, that are beneficial for brain health.

You can help your child overcome food neophobia by rethinking how you introduce new foods. Remember, kids are more likely to eat foods that are familiar.

So, your goal is to make a food more familiar. To do this, you'll want to offer a new food often in a variety of interesting ways. Regular exposure and variety are the perfect combination to help ease any fear of new foods and expand the variety of nutritious foods your child will want to try. Be creative and stick with it. You'll soon see little fingers eager to try the now familiar food.

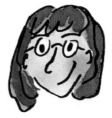

Did You Know?

Fresh fruits and vegetables are cheaper than processed forms such as canned, frozen, dried or juice.

The price per pound may seem high, but when researchers at the U.S. Department of Agriculture (USDA) compared the price per serving of 36 fruits and vegetables in both fresh and processed forms, they found that fresh was overwhelming the cheapest way to go.

Smart Moves for More Variety

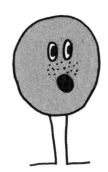

Here are 12 key strategies you can implement today to help introduce your child to new food experiences. Choose one or two to start and build from there. You'll soon be rewarded with a child who enjoys a wider variety of healthy foods to better fuel his or her active brain.

1 **Stock your home with more healthy foods.** Few habits will have more impact on what your child eats at home than your efforts to bring more healthy foods into your home, including fruits and vegetables.

2 **Make healthy choices ready-to-serve.** Don't underestimate the value of preparing foods to be at the ready when your child is looking for a snack. For example, wash grapes, cut them into small bunches and place in a bowl in the fridge. When reaching for the healthy choice requires little or no preparation on your child's part, it's likely to be the first choice.

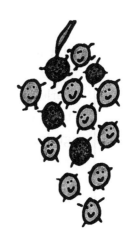

3 **Limit junk food at home.** The easiest way to curtail your child's intake of junk food at home is to avoid bringing it into your kitchen.

4 **Limit goodies to one serving at a time.** If you choose to bring a few not-so-nutritious "goodies" into your home, serve them up in single serving portions to discourage overeating. This is especially important when you purchase oversized items typically sold at warehouse club stores. The larger sizes may be friendly on your budget, but they can encourage overeating. Serve one serving and put the rest away—out of view—back in the pantry, fridge or freezer. Leaving the container in plain view tends to encourage a second or third helping.

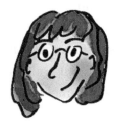

Did You Know?

We're creatures of habit—consuming the same foods day in and out. But, one way to add more variety to your child's diet is with whole grains. Has your child tried barley, bran, brown rice, bulgur, cornmeal, kasha, oat bran, quinoa, wheat germ, whole wheat or other whole grains? All are excellent sources of fiber.

Why not make a trip to your local store that features these grains in bins and give one a try? Who knows, you may stumble on a healthy winner!

5 **Model healthy eating habits.** Be adventurous yourself about trying new foods. Kids notice more than you may think and are likely to try foods that their parents or older siblings enjoy.

6 **Encourage your kids to ask, "Where's the fruit or veggie?" at every meal.** Whether it's fresh, frozen, canned or juice, it all counts. If it's missing, ask what can be added to complete the meal. This habit helps your kids become comfortable with the notion that a complete meal includes at least one fruit or vegetable—banana slices on morning cereal, a crisp apple at lunch or steamed carrots at dinner.

7 **Don't overlook junk foods masquerading as healthy choices.** Foods with no nutritional value are nothing more than junk food regardless of their food group. For example, a trendy new breakfast cereal may be loaded with sugar and have a nutritional profile more like a candy bar. If these types of foods are on your kid's must-have list, treat them like any other junk food—an occasional choice rather than a daily staple.

8 **Try different textures.** Don't forget that the texture of food is especially important for children, so before giving up on introducing a new food, experiment with different textures. Your little one may pass on crisp apple slices but gobble up applesauce with a smile.

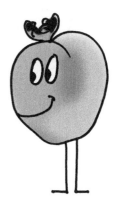

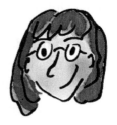

Did You Know?

Growing your own vegetables is easier than you may think when you use the square foot gardening techniques inspired by Mel Bartholomew. Thanks to a little engineering genius, he created a simple, yet elegant way to grow more in less space. Your home improvement store is sure to have all the basics to get started—planting box, seeds and soil mix.

Grab the kids and spend a few hours on a weekend afternoon mixing your soil and planting your seeds. Pick a spot where it's easy to water frequently. In a few short weeks, you'll be rewarded with a bounty of vegetables worthy of your dinner table. What's more, the kids will love watching those tiny seeds transform into ripe tomatoes, green peppers, plump zucchini and other nutritious vegetables. Need more inspiration? Visit www.squarefootgardening.com.

9 **Don't make it a big deal.** If your child turns down new foods, don't stress. Keep offering them. It may take several attempts before your child acquires a taste for it. What's more, a little reverse psychology—"Excellent, more for me!"—may be all that's needed for a change of mind.

10 **Add some fun.** Kids can be particular about the way a food looks, but adding some fun can help entice them. Draw a raisin smile on a bowl of oatmeal. Create a broccoli forest by standing the broccoli florets in mashed potatoes. Let your creativity shine to introduce new foods in a fun way.

11 **Introduce new foods with old favorites.** The "halo" effect will help link those good thoughts and feelings about favorite foods to a new food served along side it. Introduce green beans sprinkled with your child's favorite nuts such as crunchy slivers of almonds. Introduce okra in a favorite vegetable soup. Introduce whole wheat pasta with a favorite marinara sauce. Introduce almond or soy butter by spreading it on a favorite cracker.

12 **Banish the "yucky" color syndrome.** If your child has proclaimed that all foods of one color are "yucky," consider serving them with a favorite food of another color. Serve zucchini with melted cheese; celery with peanut butter; kiwi slices with a dollop of whipped cream.

> **Parent Pearl**
>
> **Once a month, we have breakfast for dinner.** I serve up the kids' favorites—cereal, toast and grapefruit; pancakes topped with maple syrup; or a tomato and cheese omelet. By switching things up, the kids learn to be creative and see that any healthy food choice is welcome at every meal.

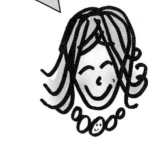

This Month's Smart Goal

I will serve at least one new fruit, vegetable or whole grain food each week.

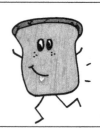

This Month's Extra Credit

I will start a "square foot" garden.

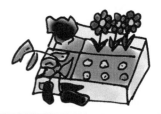

To monitor your daily progress toward your goals, use the **My Smart Tracker** forms in Chapter 14: Go for the Goal!

Part 5
Summer Fun

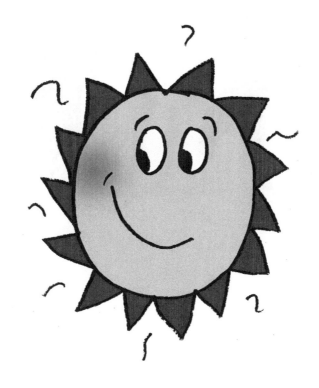

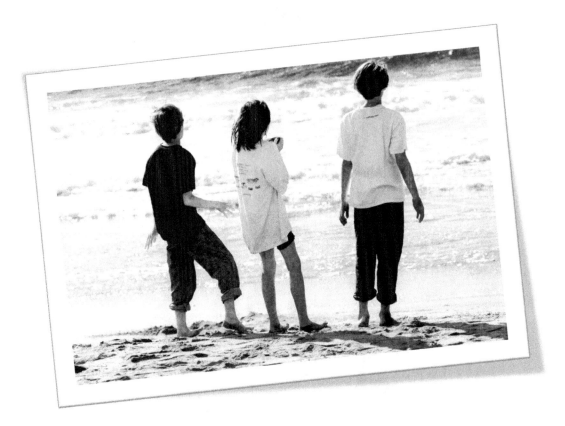

Water is the driving force of all nature.
— Leonardo da Vinci

Chapter 11

June – The Wonders of Water

It's time to welcome in the sunny days of summer, but as the temperature rises, so too does your child's need for fluid. Since staying well hydrated is essential for peak performance—both mentally and physically—there's no better time to focus on helping your child consume an adequate intake of water. If you're like most people, however, you may overlook the importance of this versatile nutrient. Not only is water essential to digest food, it's needed for lymph, the immune system fluid that helps ward off illness. Water transports nutrients throughout the body, dissipates excess heat through perspiration and eliminates toxic byproducts from the body. What's more, water is critical for the brain to function properly. In fact, most of the brain—about 75 percent—is water.

How Much Water Is Enough?

Children need between 7 and 10 cups of water daily, depending on their age and gender, according to the Institute of Medicine's Food and Nutrition Board. This recommendation includes water contained in food, beverages and drinking water.

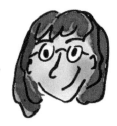

Did You Know?

While summer typically signals a break from the traditional classroom setting, it still offers many learning opportunities from taking nature hikes to visiting museums, libraries or other cultural centers. In fact, any outing can be a time to grow brain cells and make new connections.

Be sure to take full advantage of these activities, especially ones that help polish math skills. Research reveals that the first four weeks of a new school year are devoted to relearning previous material. Sadly, math skills are especially prone to decline.

To keep skills razor sharp over the summer months, consider developing a routine so that your child learns something new every day.

Recommended Water Intake	
Age	**Amount**
4 to 8 years (girls and boys)	7 cups (56 ounces)
9 to 13 years (girls)	9 cups (72 ounces)
9 to 13 years (boys)	10 cups (80 ounces)
Source: Food and Nutrition Board, Institute of Medicine	

Take a practical approach

While the Board's recommended water guidelines are good advice, they're not the most practical. A more practical approach is to encourage your child to be a scientist. Before flushing, ask your child to take a quick peek at the color of his or her urine in the toilet bowl. If it's dark – the color of apple juice – it's likely a sign of dehydration and more water is needed. If it's only slightly yellow – the color of lemonade – your child is likely well hydrated. Other signs of dehydration are smelly urine or the ability to produce only a small amount of urine.

Exceptions to the rule

There are, however, at least a few exceptions to these color and smell rules. For example, if your child recently took a multivitamin, the results may be skewed. Why? Many multivitamins contain riboflavin, a B vitamin, which can lead to bright yellow urine. Likewise, eating beets will produce urine with a reddish hue. In addition, some people who eat asparagus report that they have very smelly urine—it's normal and depends on their genetic makeup. Researchers have yet to pinpoint the exact reason for this pungent mystery. It may be because some people are better able to digest certain compounds in asparagus into more odor-causing byproducts that are excreted in urine. Or, they may have a more finely tuned sense of smell that's better at detecting the stinky stuff. Either way, it only takes one serving of the tender green stalks for your child to know whether they belong to the stinker group.

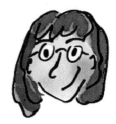

Did You Know?

Dehydration is the most preventable sports injury. Consider weighing your child before and after a sports event. For every pound lost, make sure your child drinks at least 16 ounces (2 cups) of water to adequately replenish replenish fluid lost in sweat.

Drink Up to Avoid Sports Injury

Getting enough water is critical if you have a sports girl or boy. The combination of exertion and heat can cause a decrease in performance, but more importantly, it can be harmful to your child's overall health. The American College of Sports Medicine has teamed up with like-minded groups to sponsor a public safety program called "Defeat the Heat." This program encourages parents and coaches to teach young athletes to "Think, bring, drink, and check" to avoid dehydration—the most preventable of all sports injuries. You can easily help your active child stay properly hydrated by following these four "Defeat the Heat" rules:

- Think of fluids as part of your child's essential safety equipment.
- Bring the right kinds of fluids to practices and competitions.
- Drink before, during and after activity.
- Check hydration status by monitoring the color of urine.

Parent Pearl

I look for fun ways to practice math skills with my kids during our regular routine. We track and chart the daily temperature. When driving, I give the kids math challenges or ask them to read a map. When shopping, I ask them how much change we should get back. It's a great way to keep their skills sharp.

Sports Drinks: Best & Worst

Hands down, the best drink for everyday hydration is water. However, if your child is exercising or playing a competitive sport that lasts more than one hour, then some of the commercial electrolyte drink options may be a better bet. These beverages help replenish electrolytes, such as sodium and potassium, and vitamins, such as the B vitamins, that are lost in excess sweat or that are needed in greater amounts.

Taste counts

If your child just doesn't like water, try offering a lightly flavored beverage. Research suggests that the added flavor may encourage your child to drink more and stay better hydrated.

Cool counts

At one time, it was thought that cold beverages leave the stomach faster. That's not the case. However, a cold beverage can affect the perception of body heat, which means your child is likely to feel cooler after drinking a cool one.

Say, "No!" to soft drinks

Soft drinks are nothing more than liquid sugar that fill your child's diet with empty calories. Unfortunately, kids—and teens—are now drinking soda with alarming frequency, and it's slowly crowding out calcium-rich milk as their beverage of choice. In fact, over the 25-year period from 1977 to 2002, soda intake among children, aged 6 to 11 years, jumped over 30 percent, while milk intake declined about 20 percent, based on national food survey data from the United States Department of Agriculture (USDA). In practical terms, the increase translates into a daily soda intake, on average, of about 15 ounces for children in this age group. For teens, the increase was even higher— equivalent to a daily intake of soda, on average, of 25 ounces.

Is Tap Water So Terrible?

Many people choose bottle water because they believe it's safe and purer than tap water; others claim taste and convenience are most important. However, one of the most common reasons people turn the tap off and reach for the bottle is the perception that bottled water is a safer option. To better understand how accurate—or inaccurate—this perception is, it helps to know how the two products are regulated. Bottled water is considered a food and, thus, is regulated by the U.S. Food and Drug Administration (FDA). Tap water, by contrast, is regulated by the U.S. Environmental Protection Agency (EPA). Both varieties may contain contaminates such as bacteria, arsenic, lead or pesticides, but both also undergo testing to confirm contamination, if any, is low enough to be considered safe. Most healthy adults can tolerate exposure to trace amounts of these contaminants. Children and other groups, however, may be sensitive to even low levels of contaminants. To learn more about the purity of the tap water in your area, visit the EPA's website at www.epa.gov/safewater/dwinfo/index.html.

A Primer on Plastic

When it comes to plastic containers, you'll want to know the recycling code for safe use. It's the number on the bottom of the container that corresponds to the type of plastic. There are seven codes. Numbers 1, 2, 4 and 5 are considered relatively safe—although number 1 is good only for one time use, so don't refill. The others (3, 6 and 7) are still under review. For now, here are the basics for safe use:

1 **Sniff and taste.** If there's a hint of plastic odor or taste in your water, don't drink it.

2 **Keep bottled water away from the heat.** This helps prevent chemicals from leaching into the water.

3 **Don't reuse bottles intended for single use.** They are a potential breeding ground for harmful bacteria.

4 **Use suitable containers.** Choose rigid, reusable containers. For hot or acidic liquids, choose thermoses with stainless steel or ceramic interiors.

Cost-Saving Filter Options

If you like the taste and the quality of bottled water, but want more bang for your buck, consider the cost-saving value of high-quality water filters.

Water purified with these products generally costs less than buying bottled water. According to one manufacturer, its high-end faucet filter system provides water for 18 cents a gallon, a big savings from the $1 or more that's typically charged for an 8- to 12-ounce bottle of water.

Experts report that consumers can feel confident about the water quality provided by these brand name home-filtration systems. However, a word to the wise: Make sure that you follow the manufacturer's instructions. Without proper maintenance, it's possible that bacteria or other contaminants can build up in the products.

Parent Pearl

When my daughter says, "I'm hungry, mommy," I always offer water first. Since much of hunger is actually thirst, it's an easy way to help make sure she stays properly hydrated.

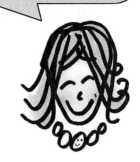

The Caffeine Scoop

Caffeine is a diuretic that increases the body's ability to expel water. This diuretic effect, in turn, leads to dehydration in your child. Thus, kids should limit their caffeine intake. In fact, there really is no need to introduce caffeinated foods or beverages into your child's diet. We suggest that you avoid them or limit their use. As a practical rule: Less is best. The U.S. government has yet to provide caffeine guidelines for kids; however, the Canadian government provides age-based guidelines that can serve as general guidance for a "less is best" approach:

Canadian Caffeine Guidelines for Children	
Age	**Daily Caffeine Limit**
4 to 6 years	45 milligrams or less
7 to 9 years	63 milligrams or less
10 to 12 years	85 milligrams or less
Source: Health Canada. Caffeine in Food. Available at: http://www.hc-sc.gc.ca.	

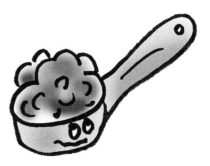

Where Does Caffeine Hide?

Coffee isn't the only food with caffeine. In fact, it shows up in a wide variety of foods that may be a part of your child's regular diet. Here are a few of the more common foods with hidden caffeine:

Caffeine Content of Select Foods and Beverages	
Food or Beverage	**Caffeine**
Coffee, 6 fluid ounces	103 milligrams
Soda, cola types, 12 fluid ounces	11-70 milligrams
Soda, Mountain Dew®, 12 fluid ounces*	55 milligrams
Soda, pepper types, 12 fluid ounces	37 milligrams
Tea, brewed, 6 fluid ounces	36 milligrams
Chocolate, dark, 1 ounce	27 milligrams
Chocolate, semi-sweet, 1 ounce	18 milligrams
Nestle® Crunch®, 1 bar (1.4 ounces)	10 milligrams
Chocolate powder, 2 to 3 heaping teaspoons	8 milligrams
Chocolate Milk, 8 ounces	8 milligrams
Chocolate syrup, 2 tablespoons	5 milligrams
Cocoa mix, 1 ounce packet	5 milligrams
Hershey's® Mr. Goodbar®, 1.75 ounces	5 milligrams

* Most non-cola carbonated beverages contain no caffeine.
Source: *Bowes & Church's Food Values of Portions Commonly Used.* 17th ed.
JB Lippincott Company: Philadelphia, Pa; 1998.

8 Brain Boosters for Summer Days

If you need some inspiration for fun activities to challenge your child's mental skills over the summer, read on for eight sure-to-please options to consider:

1 **Read, read and read some more.** If you are taking a vacation or visiting a new city or other destination, research the trip ahead of time with your child. It's sure to build excitement and anticipation. Whether your plans include crossing the Panama Canal, hiking the trails at Yosemite or simply catching the tadpoles at the local park, reading about and researching the experience together ahead of time will make it come alive.

2 **Word morph.** Pick a three-letter word and change one letter at a time. Take turns and see how many different words you can come up with. Dog to dig to big to rig to rip to tip. You get the idea.

3 **Encourage letter writing and drawing.** To keep your child's writing skills sharp and the communication lines open, encourage letter writing to friends and relatives during the summer months. Scan and save an e-copy of the letters before sending for a great keepsake. You can also scan artwork—and other well-done school projects—to enjoy for years to come.

Parent Pearl

I've become a scanning guru thanks to my daughter's love of drawing. I want to preserve her work, so when a new masterpiece is ready, I scan it right away and save to an e-file. It's a great way to preserve these treasures to enjoy for years to come.

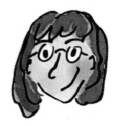

Did You Know?

One of the best resources for the freshest fruits and vegetables for your table is your community's farmers market. It's a win-win situation. You support your local farmers, and they deliver peak nutrition. To find a list of farmers markets near you, visit the Local Harvest website at www.localharvest.org.

4 **The newspaper sleuth.** Make a list of age-appropriate questions with answers that can be found in the daily newspaper.

5 **Take an alphabet walk.** Enjoy a walk together and take turns finding objects in the alphabet: ant, bee, concrete, dirt and so on.

6 **Zany alliterations.** Molly Magee makes marvelous mud pies. Consider starting with the letter A and then try the letter B. Have fun and be wacky!

7 **Fictionary.** Pick an obscure word from the dictionary and write down its meaning. Have others write a definition as well. Read out the various definitions. Award one point to the person who gets the answer correct, award one point to the person who made up a definition that fooled the others and award one point to each person stumped by the person who chose the word.

8 **Visit the local library.** Take a trip to your local public library at least once a week. It's a community treasure—offering inexpensive access to a wide selection of books, tapes and DVDs as well as a variety of enrichment programs. Children can choose several books each week to read or have read to them.

> **Parent Pearl**
>
> **On the first day of summer vacation, the kids and I brainstorm summer activities.** We make a list of all the things we want to do during the break. We usually come up with at least 50 ideas. As we do them, we check them off. Now, I rarely hear the kids say, "I'm bored."

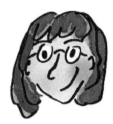

Did You Know?

If you're on snack duty for your child's sports team, choosing juicy orange slices, tangy cranberry juice and crunchy almonds will not only refuel the kids, but will provide added antioxidant protection.

This Month's Smart Goal

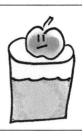

I will have my child track urine color and drink more fluid if the color resembles that of apple juice.

This Month's Extra Credit

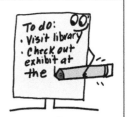

I will make a summer "To Do" list with my family of activities that stimulate both mind and body.

To monitor your daily progress toward your goals, use the **My Smart Tracker** forms in Chapter 14: Go for the Goal!

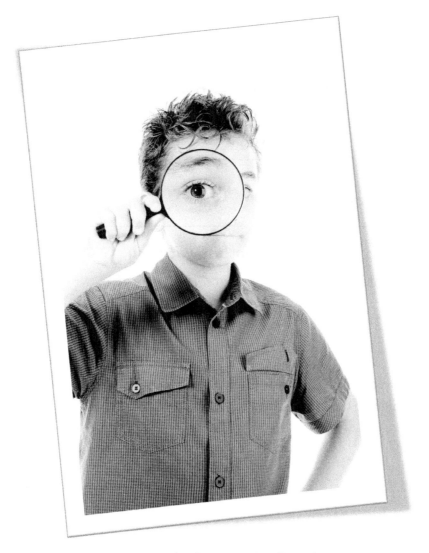

To eat is a necessity, but to eat intelligently is an art.
– *La Rochefoucauld*

Chapter 12

July – Label Reading Short Cuts

Let's face it, for most time-starved parents, grocery shopping falls into the "I can't do it fast enough" category. Trouble is, the typical supermarket carries over 45,000 items, according to the Food Marketing Institute—all competing for your time and attention.

When it comes to packaged foods, how can you quickly scan the shelves to spot the best picks to feed your family? It starts by following a few smart label reading rules that you'll learn in this chapter. Simply apply these basics as you navigate your shopping cart down the grocery aisles, and you'll be able to spot healthy foods faster than you may think.

Remember, all foods can fit into a healthy, balanced diet. That's right, all foods. In fact, research shows that banishing foods from your child's diet tends to backfire, making those forbidden no-nos even more appealing. A better choice is to use your label reading skills to separate packaged foods into two categories: the healthy, brain-building foods to enjoy regularly and the less-than-nutritious foods to consume only occasionally, if at all. Let's get started.

All facts, no puffery

Every time you pick up a new packaged food, get into the habit of finding the Nutrition Facts panel. For the most part, it's a white box with black text buried on a side or back panel of all packaged foods.

Why focus on this little gem? While marketers can extol the virtues of their products elsewhere on the label, they must follow precise rules required by the U.S. Food & Drug Administration (FDA) for what information they include in the Nutrition Facts panel. In other words, the Nutrition Facts panel is off limits to marketing puffery, making it your best resource for accurate nutrition information to make healthy food choices.

The FDA not only has strict rules about what kind of information can be included in the Nutrition Facts panel, but also controls how it looks. No enticing bold colors, splashy copy or perky cartoon characters are permitted here. In fact, compared to the marketing glitz and glamour elsewhere on food labels, the Nutrition Facts panel is downright boring. But don't be fooled, it's filled with a wealth of information about what's in a food—and what's not. The trick is knowing what to look for and how to use it to choose the healthiest foods for your child's active brain. That brings us to our nine essential label reading rules to help you quickly spot brain-building foods to buy and brain-draining foods to leave on the shelf.

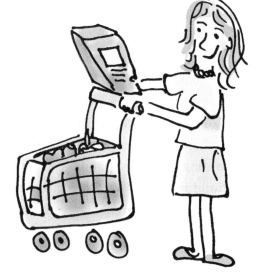

Rule 1: A Serving Is Not a Portion

The serving size is the most important information in the Nutrition Facts panel. In fact, it's so important that the FDA requires food manufacturers to prominently display it at the top of the panel, making it especially easy to spot on packaged foods.

Why is the serving size so important? All other information in the Nutrition Facts panel—all of it—is based on serving size. If you overlook it and jump right to scanning information about calories, fat and other nutrients, you will likely grossly overestimate or underestimate what your child is actually consuming.

Using the serving size, you need only apply a little light math to determine the real portion size your child truly eats and, more importantly, the amount of nutrients he or she is actually consuming.

Servings, portions and handfuls

Most kids love potato chips, and most parents offer them as an occasional indulgence. Potato chips are also a great example of just how different a serving size on a food label can be from the real-world portion your child eats.

Grab a bag and take a quick look at the Nutrition Facts panel. You'll see that regular potato chips are typically labeled for a serving size of about 1 ounce regardless of whether you're buying the oversized bag from your local warehouse club store or a single-serving bag (see example on next page).

In practical terms, each 1-ounce serving is about a handful of potato chips or about 20 chips. But if two handfuls, or about 40 chips, is more typical of the portion your child eats, you'll need to double the amount of calories, fat and other nutrients listed in the Nutrition Facts panel for a more accurate measure of what your child is really eating.

Look here for serving size

Nutrition Facts

Serving Size 20 Chips (1oz or 28g)

Amount per Serving

Calories 150   Calories from Fat 90

	% Daily Value*
Total Fat 10g	15%
Saturated Fat 1g	5%
Monounsaturated Fat 6g	
Polyunsaturated Fat 3g	
Trans Fat 0g	
Cholesterol 0mg	0%
Sodium 180mg	8%
Total Carbohydrate 15g	5%
Dietary Fiber 1g	4%
Sugars 0g	
Protein 2g	4%

*Percent Daily Values are based on a 2,000 calorie diet.

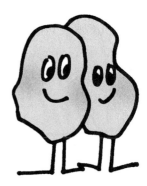

How many servings are in your portion?

Here's a great exercise to better understand the difference between a typical portion and the serving size listed on a packaged food. The next time you offer your child potato chips, count out the number of chips you actually put on the plate. Really, count them out. Now, check the label to see how close your portion is to the serving size listed in the Nutrition Facts panel. Is it closer to 20 chips (one serving), 40 chips (two servings) or more? If you're like most, your typical portion is likely to be two, three or more servings.

Remember, all foods can be part of a healthy, balanced diet, but controlling portion size, especially for those less-than-nutrition foods, will allow some wiggle room for small indulgences while helping to ensure that your child fills up on brain-building foods and maintains a healthy weight.

Rule 2: Every Calories Counts

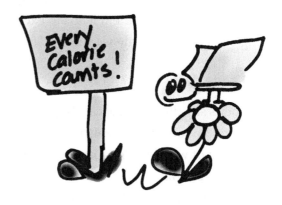

Another key listing in the Nutrition Facts panel is calories per serving. Now that you're portion-size savvy, you can use the calorie information to accurately estimate how much a packaged food contributes to your child's daily needs.

Just how many calories does your child need to maintain a healthy body weight? It really depends on age, activity level and gender. On average, younger kids, aged 4 to 8 years, need between 1,200 and 2,000 calories per day to maintain a healthy body weight. Sedentary children—those who get less than 30 minutes of moderate physical activity on most days—have calorie needs on the low end of the range at about 1,200 to 1,4000 calories per day. On the other hand, active kids—those who get the equivalent of a brisk three-mile walk every day—require a calorie intake on the high end of the range or about 1,400 to 2,000 calories per day.

The total calorie needs for older kids, age 9 to 13 years, are similar or higher, but the same activity rule applies: Active kids need more calories than their sedentary counterparts to maintain a healthy body weight.

To find more details about the calories needs for your child see **Recommended Daily Intake: Calories** in Chapter 15: Tables, Tips & More.

Rule 3: Wiggle, But Just A Little

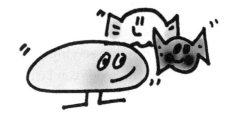

Every diet deserves a little wiggle room for potato chips, cookies, and other less-than-nutritious, but oh-so-yummy foods. In fact, nutrition experts report there's no reason a healthy diet can't include a few empty calories.

The trick is to include just enough empty calories to satisfy a craving, but not so much that filling up on them leads to excess weight gain or prevents your child from eating enough nutrient-dense foods to fuel the body and brain.

What's the daily limit?

Experts say diets with about 10 percent of daily calories from empty calories would still be considered healthy. So, depending on your child's age and activity, the amount of wiggle room for empty calories is in the range of 120 calories to about 260 calories per day.

This may seem like plenty of calories for a splurge, but they can add up fast when your child is reaching for high-fat or sugar-laden processed foods. Think of a typical 12-ounce can of soda; it packs about 160 calories and can easily meet a child's daily limit for empty calories.

Whether the calories your child consumes are from nutrient-dense, healthy foods or empty calories, one fact remains true: Every calorie counts.

Rule 4: Choose Fat like Goldilocks

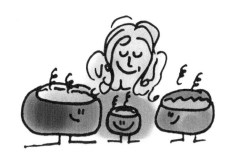

For children, 4 years of age and older, tweens and teenagers, take the Goldilocks approach to total fat intake—not too little, not too much, but just the right amount for growing bodies and active brains. What is the "right" amount of fat for your child? According to the *Dietary Guidelines for Americans*, a healthy fat intake for these ages is about 25 percent to 35 percent of total daily calories.

Simplify with the law of averages

How should you choose packaged foods to meet this guideline? The simplest way is to use the law of averages. With a little math, you can calculate the percent calories from fat for any packaged food. Then, you can choose more packaged foods that are lower in fat (i.e., no more than 35 percent calories from fat) and fewer foods that are higher in fat (i.e., more than 35 percent calories from fat).

Where do you start?

The Nutrition Facts panel is the place to start. It not only prominently displays total calories, but also lists calories from fat, when a food contains fat. To calculate percent fat, find the "Calories from Fat" entry and divide by the "Calories" entry. Multiply by 100 to convert your answer to percent calories from fat.

Practice makes perfect

As an example, take a look at the Nutrition Facts panel for graham crackers on the next page. You can see that one cracker—the two-square rectangle variety—has a total of 60 calories ("Calories 60") and 12 calories from fat ("Calories from Fat 12"). So, it has 20 percent calories from fat, making graham crackers a low-fat snack.

Cookies and crackers are snack favorites for kids, and any brand—in the right portion—can be part of a healthy diet. Simply choose lower fat options more often than higher fat options. For example, Fig Newtons®—with less than 20 percent fat calories—would be a good choice for regular snacks. By contrast, Oreo® cookies—with almost 40 percent fat calories—are best consumed only occasionally.

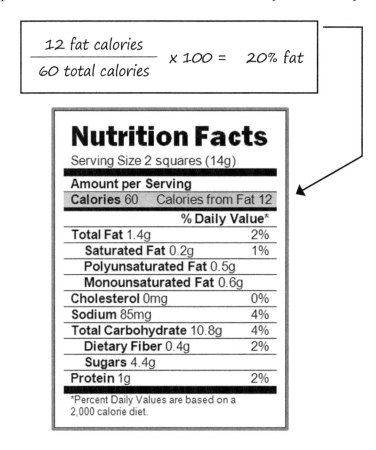

$$\frac{12 \text{ fat calories}}{60 \text{ total calories}} \times 100 = 20\% \text{ fat}$$

Nutrition Facts

Serving Size 2 squares (14g)

Amount per Serving

Calories 60   Calories from Fat 12

	% Daily Value*
Total Fat 1.4g	2%
Saturated Fat 0.2g	1%
Polyunsaturated Fat 0.5g	
Monounsaturated Fat 0.6g	
Cholesterol 0mg	0%
Sodium 85mg	4%
Total Carbohydrate 10.8g	4%
Dietary Fiber 0.4g	2%
Sugars 4.4g	
Protein 1g	2%

*Percent Daily Values are based on a 2,000 calorie diet.

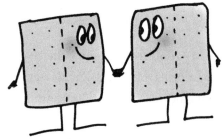

Rule 5: Avoid Brain-Draining Fats

The Nutrition Facts panel on food labels is also a wealth of information about the types of fats found in packaged foods. In fact, the FDA requires manufacturers of all packaged foods to list both the amount and type of fats in the Nutrition Facts panel. You'll find up to four types of fats listed: saturated, monounsaturated, polyunsaturated and trans fats.

The troublesome duo

While all four types of fat contain nine calories per gram, two types are especially detrimental to growing brains: saturated fats and trans fats.

Why? Diets high in saturated fats can lead to high blood cholesterol that can clog the blood vessels that nourish the brain. Trans fats deliver a double whammy to the brain. Not only do they raise artery-clogging blood cholesterol, but trans fats can worm their way into cell membranes where they wreak havoc with the membrane's ability to remain pliable and flexible. In short, trans fats lead to more rigid cell membranes that limit the ability of brain cells to take up valuable nutrients, expel metabolic byproducts and perform at their best.

Food sources of saturated fats

The main sources of saturated fats are foods from animals and a few plants. For example, beef, beef fat, veal, lamb, pork, lard, chicken fat, butter, cream, milk, cheese and other dairy products contain saturated fats.

Plant foods that contain saturated fats include the so-called tropical oils—coconut, coconut oil, palm oil and palm kernel oil—and cocoa butter. Another common source of saturated fats in the diet is hydrogenated vegetable oils such as margarine, shortening, cooking oils and the foods made from them.

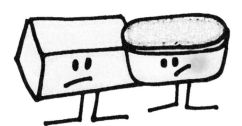

Look here for brain-draining
saturated and trans fats

Nutrition Facts

Serving Size 2 Tbsp (24g)

Amount per Serving

Calories 100   Calories from Fat 40

	% Daily Value*
Total Fat 4.5g	7%
Saturated Fat 1.5g	8%
Trans Fat 1g	
Sodium 55mg	2%
Potassium 60mg	2%
Total Carbohydrate 14g	5%
Dietary Fiber <1g	3%
Sugars 12g	
Protein 0g	2%

*Percent Daily Values are based on a
2,000 calorie diet.

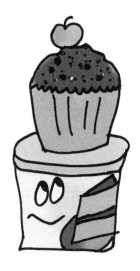

Food sources of trans fats

The manufacturing process of hydrogenation also produces trans fats, the second type of fat that can clog arteries and harm brain cells. This process changes the chemical composition of a vegetable oil to allow it to be solid at room temperature, which is an ideal texture for a wide variety of processed foods such as crackers, biscuits, doughnuts, cookies and muffins. In fact, the partially hydrogenated vegetable oils found in processed foods are the source of most—about 75 percent—of the harmful trans fat in the American diet. As an example, see the Nutrition Facts panel for a typical ready-made frosting on page 202.

Terrible with a capital "T"

Trans fats are so harmful, nutrition experts recommend you avoid them completely or at least limit them to no more than 1 percent of daily calories. For kids—and adults—this means no more than 1 to 3 grams of trans fats per day, depending on calorie needs. Yet, the typical American diet contains, on average, almost 6 grams of trans fats per day. In short, a healthy diet doesn't have much wiggle room for the added trans fats found in many processed and fast foods, so it's especially important to accurately read labels to choose products that are free of these brain-draining fats.

Parent Pearl

I use olive oil when cooking. I drizzle it on veggies, mix with balsamic vinegar for bread dipping or add a touch to noodles. It's a great tasting healthier option.

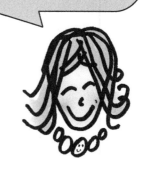

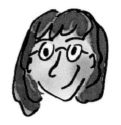

Did You Know?

Trans fats lurk in many foods that may be on your child's list of favorites. Here are just a few:

Cake (from mix)	Muffins
Candy	Pancake mix
Chicken nuggets	Pie crusts
Chocolate drink mix	Pizza dough
Cookies	Popcorn, microwave
Corn chips	Popcorn, packaged
Crackers	Potato chips
Doughnuts	Stick margarine
French fries	Taco shells (hard)
Frosting (ready-made)	Tortilla chips
Hamburger buns	Vegetable shortening

Source: U.S. Department of Agriculture

Rule 6: Choose More Low-Sodium Foods

Kids—and adults—who eat a typical American diet tend to consume too much sodium, which can send blood pressure racing skyward and increase the risk of heart disease and kidney disease. You can help keep your child's intake of sodium in a healthy range using your label reading skills. After all, processed and packaged foods top the list of high-sodium foods in the American diet. Focus on these culprits, and you're sure to make a big dent in your child's sodium intake. Healthy habits described in other chapters—eating more fruits and veggies, maintaining a healthy body weight and staying active—also help keep blood pressure in the health range.

Just how much sodium is considered healthy?

Experts recommend that young kids, age 4 to 8 years, consume an amount of sodium in the range of 1,200 to 1,900 milligrams per day, while older kids, 9 to 13 years, should aim for an intake between 1,500 to 2,200 milligrams per day. In practical terms, that's only about ½ to 1 teaspoon of salt—much less than what kids are actually consuming. In fact by age 4, the average salt intake is a whopping 4,700 milligrams per day, according to recent research. The average intake increases with age and, by age 18, reaches 6,800 milligrams per day. And, that's not including salt added in cooking or at the table.

Look beyond the salt shaker

Sodium isn't just in the salt shaker. In fact, any substance with sodium in the name, such as monosodium glutamate (MSG), bisodium carbonate or sodium nitrite, is the same sodium found in sodium chloride or table salt. To quickly find the sodium content of packaged foods, look in the Nutrition Facts panel. And, since the sodium content of similar packaged foods can vary by several hundred milligrams, the Nutrition Facts panel is an ideal tool to compare products to choose the lower sodium option.

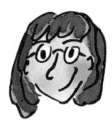

Did You Know?

Some sensitive people may experience flushing, nausea, headaches or itching when they consume foods with monosodium glutamate, commonly known as MSG.

Another option is to look for packaged products with front-of-package claims such as "low sodium" or "very low sodium." The FDA limits the use of the term "low sodium" to packaged foods with no more than 140 milligrams of sodium per serving (5% Daily Value). The term "very low sodium" has stricter guidelines and is limited to packaged foods with no more than 35 milligrams of sodium per serving (1% Daily Value).

As a rule, always double check the Nutrition Facts panel for a food with front-of-package claims such as "salt-free," "unsalted," or "without added salt." The FDA regulates these terms as well but they only mean no salt is added during processing. The salt content of the food may still be high from naturally occurring sodium or other sodium-containing additives.

Using your sodium know-how

Test your label reading skills on two kid-friendly foods that are notorious for being high in sodium: soup and hard pretzels. During your next trip to the grocery store, take a look at both regular and low-sodium varieties. You just may be amazed at the dramatic difference in sodium content.

For example, choose a regular tomato soup, and you could be serving up over 700 milligrams of sodium (30% Daily Value). Switch to a low-sodium variety, and you can cut the sodium to 50 milligrams per serving (2% Daily Value). As an example, see the Nutrition Facts panels for regular and low-sodium tomato soup on page 208.

Apply the same strategy to choosing a brand of hard pretzels, and you can cut the sodium content from over 800 milligrams per serving (34% Daily Value) in the salted variety to under 200 milligrams per serving (7% Daily Value) for an unsalted version.

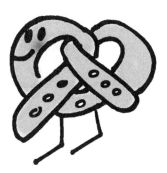

Every little change adds up to big savings, so start applying your label reading skills today.

Look here to compare
the sodium content of foods

Nutrition Facts

Serving Size About 1 cup (7¼ oz)

Amount per Serving	
Calories 130 Calories from Fat 30	

	% **Daily Value***
Total Fat 3g	5%
Saturated Fat 1.5g	8%
Trans Fat 0g	
Cholesterol 5mg	2%
Sodium 50mg	2%
Total Carbohydrate 23g	8%
Dietary Fiber 3g	12%
Sugars 17g	
Protein 2g	

*Percent Daily Values are based on a 2,000 calorie diet.

Nu

Servi

Amou

Calor

Total Fat 1g	2%
Saturated Fat 0.5g	3%
Trans Fat 0g	
Cholesterol < 5mg	2%
Sodium 720mg	30%
Total Carbohydrate 21g	7%
Dietary Fiber 3g	12%
Sugars 8g	
Protein 1g	

*Percent Daily Values are based on a 2,000 calorie diet.

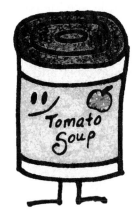

Rule 7: Know the Sweet Lingo

Sugars naturally occur in fruits, grains, milk and milk products, but sugars are also added to packaged foods for a variety of reasons. These added sugars impart a sweet taste to foods and, in many foods, can help improve the texture and appearance. Trouble is, consuming too much of these added sugars can sap your child's brain power and increase their risk for other health concerns.

The Nutrition Facts panel provides information on total sugars per serving, but does not distinguish between sugars that are naturally present in foods and added sugars. For that, you'll need to look to the Ingredients panel, which is found on food labels right below the Nutrition Facts panel. Common terms for added sugar are listed below. Look for these terms in the Ingredients panel, and notice where they are placed in the list of ingredients. The FDA requires manufacturers to list ingredients in descending order by weight. For example, if sugar—or another term for added sugar—is listed among the first three ingredients, the food is likely high in added sugar. As an example, see the Nutrition Facts panel for granola on page 211.

Common Terms For Added Sugar in Packaged Foods		
Brown sugar	Glucose	Malt syrup
Corn sweetener	High-fructose corn syrup	Molasses
Corn syrup	Honey	Raw sugar
Dextrose	Invert sugar	Sucrose
Fructose	Lactose	Sugar
Fruit juice concentrates	Maltose	Syrup

A word about sugar alcohols

Mannitol, sorbitol, xylitol and other sugar alcohols are popular sweeteners for special dietary foods. These ingredients are produced commercially from various sugars. Sugar alcohols are more slowly absorbed from the digestive tract than sugar, which makes them a good choice for special dietary foods. They also tend to be less likely to cause tooth decay. However, when consumed in large amounts, sugar alcohols can have a laxative effect and cause digestive upset in sensitive people, which limits their use in foods.

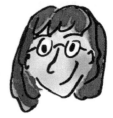

Did You Know?

The ingredients in packaged foods are always listed in an Ingredients panel right below the Nutrition Facts panel.

What's more, ingredients are always listed in descending order by weight. So, the amounts of ingredients at the top of the list are more than those at the bottom of the list.

Nutrition Facts

Serving Size 2/3 Cup (55g)

Amount per Serving

Calories 210   Calories from Fat 25

% Daily Value*

Total Fat 3g	5%
Saturated Fat 1.5g	7%
Trans Fat 0g	
Monounsaturated Fat 0.5g	
Polyunsaturated Fat 0.5g	
Cholesterol 0mg	0%
Sodium 135mg	6%
Total Carbohydrate 45g	15%
Dietary Fiber 3g	12%
Sugars 18g	
Protein 4g	

*Percent Daily Values are based on a 2,000-calorie diet.

Look here for the amount of sugars

This granola has plenty of sugars, starting with the third ingredient for a total of 18 grams or 4½ teaspoons per serving.

Ingredients: Whole grain rolled oats, whole grain rolled wheat, sugar, raisins, crisp rice (rice, sugar, salt, barley malt), corn flakes (corn, sugar, salt, barley malt, corn syrup), puffed rice, whey, molasses, glycerin, coconut oil, almonds, whey protein concentrate, honey, salt, dried coconut, cinnamon, soy lecithin.

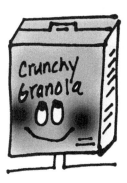

Rule 8: Focus on High-Fiber Foods

Children need high-fiber foods to keep their digestion and elimination in tip-top shape—which means fewer visits to the pediatrician. High-fiber foods not only help promote heart health, but also help control blood sugar. What's more, this versatile nutrient offers an added bonus for overweight kids. How? High-fiber foods are filling, so kids eat less, but still feel satisfied.

You'll find fiber in plant-based foods such as fruits, vegetables, dried beans and peas, nuts and whole grains. This wide variety of choices makes it even easier to include at least one high-fiber food at every meal.

How much is enough?

Just how much fiber do children need? As a rule of thumb, kids—and adults—should consume 14 grams of fiber for every 1,000 calories they eat. Younger kids, 4 to 8 years old, should aim for about 25 grams per day, while older kids, 9 to 13 years old, should aim for about 26 to 31 grams of fiber daily.

Look for "5" for high-fiber foods

When it comes to packaged foods, you can quickly find the fiber content. If the food contains enough fiber worth mentioning, you'll find it prominently listed in the Nutrition Facts panel. And, if a packaged food contains at least 5 grams of fiber per serving—that's 20 percent of the Daily Value—it's earned the right to be called "high-fiber." In this case, you're likely to also see a big, bold banner across the front of the package extolling the high-fiber virtues of the product. What's more, many supermarkets are starting to use more shelf signs to help you quickly find these nutritious choices.

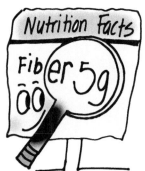

Look here for dietary fiber. Foods with 5 grams or more per serving like a hearty bean soup are high in fiber.

Nutrition Facts

Serving Size 1 cup (250 g)

Amount per Serving

Calories 160   Calories from Fat 35

	% Daily Value*
Total Fat 4g	6%
Saturated Fat 0.5g	3%
Trans Fat 0g	
Cholesterol 0g	0%
Sodium 340mg	14%
Total Carbohydrate 24g	8%
Dietary Fiber 8g	32%
Sugars 5g	
Protein 7g	

*Percent Daily Values are based on a 2,000 calorie diet.

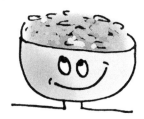

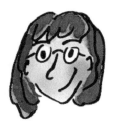

Did You Know?

One way to determine if your child is consuming enough fiber is to check stool consistency. In practical terms, simply have your child look at his or her poop. If it's a floater, it's a good indication of an adequate fiber intake. If it's a sinker, it's a sign that your child needs to eat more fiber-rich foods.

Rule 9: Not All Organic Products Are Alike

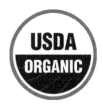

If you're interested in choosing organic foods for your family, then you'll want to keep an eye out for packaged foods with the USDA Organic Seal. The U.S. Department of Agriculture (USDA) allows manufacturers to use this seal on packaging when foods are made with 100 percent organic ingredients. However, the USDA also allows three other types of organic label claims for foods that have some—but not all—organic ingredients.

The four levels of "organic"

Here's the breakdown of the USDA's organic claims permitted for use on foods:

- **100% Organic.** Just as the claim suggests, these foods are completely organic and qualify to use the USDA Organic Seal.
- **Organic.** The contents of foods with this claim must be at least 95 percent organic by weight, excluding water and salt. These foods also qualify to use the USDA Organic Seal.
- **Made With Organic.** At least 70 percent of the contents of foods with this claim must be organic. You'll likely find the "Made with Organic" claim splashed across the front of the package, but the USDA Organic Seal is not permitted on these foods.
- **Less than 70 percent of content is organic.** Foods that meet this criterion may only list ingredients that are organic in the Ingredient panel. These foods are not permitted to mention organic on the main panel and may not display the USDA Organic Seal.

> **Parent Pearl**
>
> **We search for "the Seal."** While grocery shopping, I make a game out of seeing how many products my kids can spot with the USDA Organic Seal. It's a fun way to learn about organic foods.

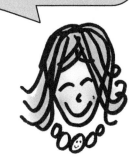

Organic animal foods

Meats, eggs and dairy products may be labeled organic when producers follow a few key rules. First, producers must allow the animals outside. Second, they cannot give the animals growth hormones or antibiotics. Finally, they must use animal feed that is organic and free of any parts of other slaughtered animals.

Parent Pearl

When it comes to milk, I only buy brands from cows not treated with hormones. I can quickly compare products by looking for the claim, "Not from cows treated with rBST." Most brands display it right on the front of the package, making it easy to compare.

This Month's Smart Goal

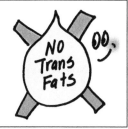

I will read the Nutrition Facts panel on packaged foods to choose brands with zero grams of trans fats.

This Month's Extra Credit

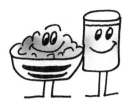

I will serve portions of packaged foods that are no more than the serving size listed on the Nutrition Facts panel.

To monitor your daily progress toward your goals, use the **My Smart Tracker** forms in Chapter 14: Go for the Goal!

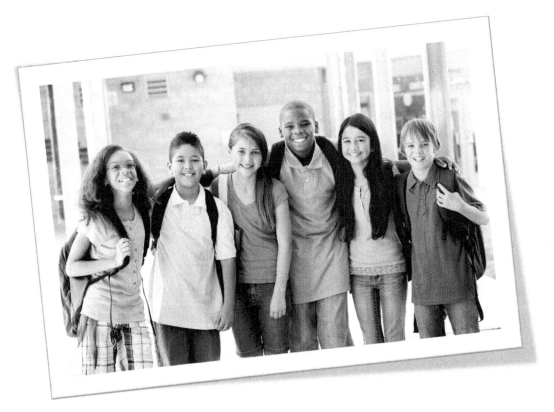

Good habits, once established
are just as hard to break as are bad habits.
— Robert Puller

Chapter 13

August – Prep for a New School Year

For most parents of young children, August means back-to-school shopping. Whether your child's school clothes are standard issue uniforms or outfits that allow more self expression, a quick inventory of last year's wardrobe is sure to confirm the inevitable: Your child has outgrown, well, just about everything.

The growth spurt that's sending you to the mall is easy to spot. You may have noticed that your child's face has matured along with a tighter jaw line and a smile that now sports more permanent teeth. It's an incredible transformation.

Even more incredible is the physical change occurring in your child's brain as the complex circuitry of dendrites, axons and other brain cells work to activate learning and memory. You can help ensure that your child's brain stays fueled and ready to learn throughout the new school year by adding a few simple items to your back-to-school shopping list and school routine. Read on to learn how.

Lunch Box Essentials

Packing a lunch becomes much easier when you have the proper supplies on hand. So, when hitting the shops to get school supplies, don't forget the following lunch essentials:

1 **Lunch box.** Young kids love getting a new lunch box with the latest cartoon character, action figure or other popular design. Whatever the choice, make sure it's both sturdy and easy to clean. Also, remember to write your child's name in it—using a permanent marker—in case it gets lost on the playground.

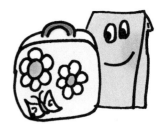

2 **Cold packs.** Cold packs are a must. It only takes a few hours for a non-refrigerated lunch to start growing harmful bacteria that can cause food-borne illnesses. What's more, chilled foods allowed to sit at room temperature tend to go straight to the trash. Warm string cheese, anyone? Consider purchasing several cold packs to ensure you always have one in the freezer ready for use. Some even come in fun shapes—such as soccer balls, baseballs and flowers.

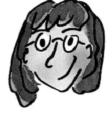

Did You Know?

The Centers for Disease Control and Prevention (CDC) provides an interactive tool called "Analyze My Plate." With a click of the mouse, your computer-savvy child can design a healthy meal or analyze his or her breakfast—or any meal, for that matter. This free tool is available at www.fruitsandveggiesmatter.gov. Click "Interactive Tools" and then "Analyze My Plate."

3 **Thermos.** Be sure to purchase two high-quality thermoses—one for beverages and another for food. The best choices are those made from stainless steel. For food, choose a small one (about 10 ounces) with a wide mouth so that your child can see what's inside. Make sure that it can safely store hot foods for up to 6 hours.

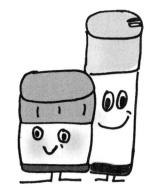

4 **Containers for sandwiches and snacks.** Sturdy containers for sandwiches and other snacks are a plus. You'll avoid overusing disposable baggies, which is friendly to both your budget and the environment.

5 **Stickers, jokes or fancy napkins.** Don't forget to pack a little fun in your child's lunch box. Keep a stash of jokes, riddles and bright stickers on hand for plenty of options to lighten the noontime meal. Be sure to mix it up to keep your child guessing—that's half the fun. It's a no-fuss way to keep your child smiling throughout the new school year.

Easing into the School Year

With the start of school only a few weeks away, consider some of the following tips to make sure your youngster gets off on the right foot.

Get organized

Place all upcoming events—ice cream socials, back-to-school nights, PTA meetings, sports events, scout functions and other activities—on a central calendar or, for the tech-savvy, in a smart phone. Organize a homework niche for your child, and double up on school supplies so that you can keep one set here.

Sweet slumber

If your child has been enjoying a more relaxed bedtime schedule during the summer months, it's time to ease back into a structured routine in preparation for school. After all, optimal learning demands an alert mind that only a good night's sleep can provide. About two weeks before the start of school, start adjusting your child's bedtime hour back to mesh with the upcoming school year. Typically, most preschoolers should sleep 10 to 12 hours per day, while older children and teens need at least 9 hours of sleep per day. That means, if your fifth grader wakes up at 6:30 a.m. during school days, aim for a bedtime—and lights out—no later than 9:00 p.m., to allow 30 minutes for sleep to set in.

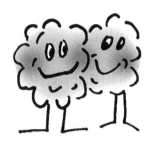

The "night before" habit

The more you can do the night before a school day, the less chaotic the morning will be. Teach your child to place everything he or she needs for the next school day by the front door. This includes homework neatly tucked inside the backpack. Also, encourage your child to layout the next day's outfit.

The afternoon snack

After long school days, your child is likely to arrive home with a rumbling stomach. An after-school snack is a great routine to help your child replenish his or her energy level after a full day of non-stop activity—both mental and physical. With a little planning, you can be prepared to offer healthy snacks. Fresh cut fruit, a quesadilla made with a whole wheat tortilla or a whole grain bagel with peanut butter are just a few snacks that will help curb hunger and refuel your child to tackle the day's homework.

Backpack Know-How

One click of the mouse will send you on your way to a whole host of credible online websites filled with expert tips about backpack safety from the American Academy of Pediatrics to the National Safety Council to the American Physical Therapy Association.

What's more, the American Occupational Therapy Association celebrates their annual National School Backpack Awareness Day on the third Wednesday in September when these hardworking ergonomic experts offer safety tips for students, parents, educators, school administrators and community members alike.

While the experts may debate about the finer points of backpack safety, all of them—yes, all of them—agree on three critical actions you must take to protect your child's health. Here's the need-to-know: choose the right backpack for your child's size, teach your child how to pack it for back comfort and, finally, encourage your child to wear it properly. Focus on these basics and your child is sure to enjoy better back comfort throughout the day and have fewer aches and pains that can distract from learning.

Six Basics For Choosing A Backpack

1 **Look for sturdy, lightweight construction.** The school year can be tough on your child's backpack. After all, it needs to survive both the daily toting of textbooks and other school supplies and the drop-and-toss style of most energetic kids. With the typical school year lasting about 180 days, all those snaps, clasps, zippers and seams take a beating, which is why choosing a sturdy, well-constructed backpack is essential. Sturdy backpacks that are also lighter in weight are the best choice, as you want the backpack itself to contribute as little weight as possible.

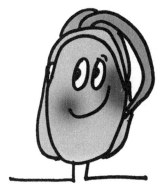

2 **Consider a trendy design.** While you're looking for a backpack that's sturdy and well-constructed, your child has an eye on one with a trendy color or design. Blend the best of both worlds by encouraging your child to be part of the decision. With so much variety in the market, you can easily select a sturdy brand that's perfectly sized for your child's height and weight in a color or design that your child prefers. The result: A sturdy backpack that your child will want to wear.

3 **Look for two shoulder straps and a waist strap.** Backpacks with two straps that are wide and padded allow your child to carry their pack across both shoulders. The result is more evenly distributed weight and more comfort. By contrast, carrying a backpack over one shoulder can lead to fatigue, poor posture and lower back pain that can stifle learning. A waist strap also helps to distribute the weight evenly, which is especially critical when the load is heavy.

4 **Choose a padded back.** A padded back certainly offers your child more comfort, but it also protects the body from pencils, pens and other sharp objects that can accidentally puncture through and cause harm.

5 **Pack smart to ease back strain.** Experts tend to agree on how to organize the contents of the backpack—place the heaviest items on the bottom, in the center and closest to the back. The debate continues, however, on how much weight your child should carry. As a general rule, children should carry backpacks that weigh no more than 10 percent to 15 percent of their body weight. Keep the load light by encouraging your child to pack only items used for the day, and get a second set of textbooks, especially heavy ones, to avoid the daily haul back and forth to school.

6 **Consider a backpack on rollers.** A backpack with rolling wheels is another option to lighten the load; however, consider how your child will use the pack. Does your child need to climb numerous stairs throughout the day with a backpack in tow? Does your child use a locker that may be too small to store a larger rolling pack? Does your child walk through snow, unpaved surfaces or other paths that may be challenging with a rolling pack? If so, a rolling backpack may not be the best choice.

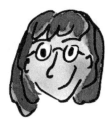

Did You Know?

Backpacks can injure more than just your child's back. According to a study published in *Pediatrics*, backpack-related injuries severe enough to send school-aged children to the emergency room also include the following:

- Foot, ankle, wrist and elbow injuries from tripping over a backpack lying on the ground.
- Head and face injuries from getting hit with a backpack.
- Shoulder and neck injuries from wearing a backpack.
- Shoulder injuries from lifting a backpack.
- Finger and other upper body injuries from taking off a backpack and reaching in.

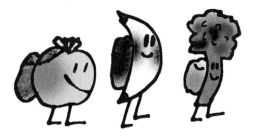

Backpack Weight Check

Fill your child's backpack for a typical school day and weigh it on a bathroom scale. Weigh your child separately. Compare your child's backpack with the recommended weight limit listed below. Is it time to lighten the load?

Your Child's Body Weight	Backpack Weight Limit (no more than)
50 lbs	5 to 7.5 lbs
55 lbs	5.5 to 8.3 lbs
60 lbs	6 to 9 lbs
65 lbs	6.5 to 9.8 lbs
70 lbs	7 to 10.5 lbs
75 lbs	7.5 to 11.3 lbs
80 lbs	8 to 12 lbs
85 lbs	8.5 to 12.8 lbs
90 lbs	9 to 13.5 lbs
95 lbs	9.5 to 14.3 lbs
100 lbs	10 to 15 lbs

Better Homework

With the official kickoff of the typical school year just a few short weeks away, August is the perfect time to prepare for the daily ritual of homework. Why? Establishing a regular routine—with an emphasis on regular—is essential to develop good study habits that are sure to help your child enjoy learning and breeze through their assignments.

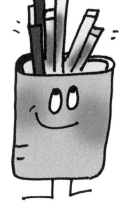

What's more, getting "homework ready" is a lot easier than you may think thanks to the experts at the American Academy of Pediatrics (AAP) who have compiled a seven-point checklist to help you establish a daily homework routine. Read on for a summary of these need-to-know basics—along with our practical tips—that are sure to help maximize your child's learning throughout the year.

1 **Establish a space for homework.** A workspace in the home that offers privacy is ideal whether it's your child's bedroom, a quiet corner of the kitchen or other part of the home. A dedicated space is ideal; but, when it's not an option, consider establishing a quiet time for the entire house, a sort of "virtual space" that is free of distractions that can disrupt homework time.

2 **Set aside plenty of time for homework.** Nothing saps effective learning like stress. By scheduling enough time to complete homework assignments without undue stress, you'll create a relaxed, calm environment that's likely to promote better learning.

3 **Establish a "house rule" to turn the TV off during homework time.** This is especially true when your child's homework space is within earshot of a noisy and distracting TV program. The bonus is scheduled quiet time for you.

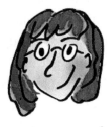

Did You Know?

Homework requires a quiet space that allows for focused attention. That's likely to be missing when kids plant themselves in the middle of a busy family room after school to break out the books.

It doesn't need to be a dedicated place, just a place without distractions. If space is limited, consider a virtual homework space during which the house is quiet. It's a great way for parents to complete their "quiet" tasks as well such as pay a few bills, read the newspaper or catch up on their paperwork.

4 **Consider a tutor for tough subjects.** If your child is having a challenge with a particular subject, consider enlisting the services of a tutor. A tutor may offer a fresh approach to learning that can help your child more easily understand a difficult subject. Discuss this option with your child's teacher who is likely to be a great resource for suggestions.

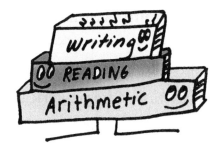

5 **Encourage your child to take regular breaks.** Regular breaks are especially important to prevent eye fatigue and neck strain, but closing the books for a few minutes and stretching also goes a long way to maintain focus and interest.

6 **Be available to answer questions and offer assistance, but avoid doing your child's homework.** This homework must-do is often easier said than done. After all, explaining a new math concept or grammar rule typically takes a bit more patience and time, but your extra effort will pay off with a child who is not only more proficient in a particular subject, but is also likely to be more confident and self-assured.

7 **Supervise computer and Internet use.** When used properly, the Internet is a great educational tool for kids. This high-tech tool offers ready access to numerous resources for school projects from point-and-click textbooks and other materials posted by teachers to interactive team projects with classmates. Trouble is, it's just as easy to navigate to the latest online game and other distractions. Keeping a watchful eye on computer time will help keep your child's focus on homework projects and away from the latest online game.

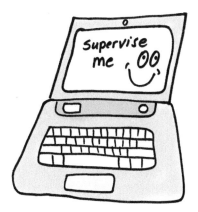

This Month's Smart Goal

At least two weeks before school starts, I will establish a homework space based on the "Better Homework" tips.

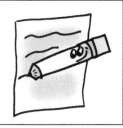

This Month's Extra Credit

At least two weeks before school starts, I will buy a backpack based on the "Backpack Know-How" tips.

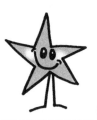

To monitor your daily progress toward your goals, use the **My Smart Tracker** forms in Chapter 14: Go for the Goal!

Part 6
Extras

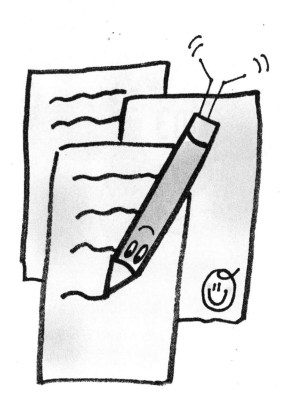

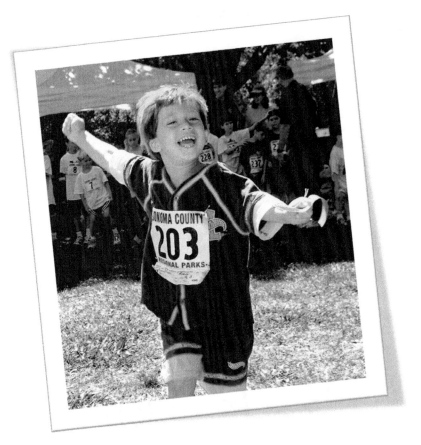

A goal properly set is halfway reached.
– Abraham Lincoln

Chapter 14

Go for the Goal!

One of the most effective ways to keep your daily motivation up as you work toward shaping the healthy habits your child needs to be smarter and healthier is to track progress. That's what this chapter is all about—fast and easy goal tracking.

Here you'll find **My Smart Tracker** forms. These pre-printed monthly tracking forms correspond to each chapter's goal and extra credit. We've also included plenty of blank forms to inspire you to track even more healthy habits.

Ready to get started? Here's how: Turn to the monthly goal you want to work on. Fill in the corresponding dates for the month. Now you're ready to track. At the end of the day, you simply grab a pen and check off whether you've made progress toward the goal.

Don't underestimate the power of this simple yet elegant tool. Few things are more motivating than seeing regular progress, especially for health-related goals.

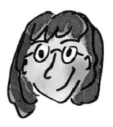

Did You Know?

Tracking your daily progress toward your SMART goals is the first step to your success. But don't forget to reflect on your monthly success.

At the end of each month, write down a short sentence or two about the progress you've made toward your monthly goal and any thoughts you may have about your success.

Seeing your progress in writing is a great confidence booster that helps keep motivation high and goals on track.

September | Goal

I will add one family meal each week
to reach at least five per week.*

*At least five is the goal, but for this goal and all others, make sure to
set them for where you and your family are. Make sure your goals are
not too hard, but not too easy either.

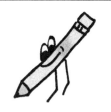

SUN	MON	TUE	WED	THU	FRI	SAT

This month I accomplished: _____

_____

_____

Notes: _____

_____

_____

September | Extra Credit

I will give my child a children's multivitamin with 18 milligrams of iron everyday, preferably at breakfast.

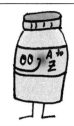

SUN	MON	TUE	WED	THU	FRI	SAT

This month I accomplished: _____
_____
_____

Notes: _____
_____
_____
_____

October | Goal

I will serve breakfast every day and include a protein-rich food.

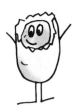

SUN	MON	TUE	WED	THU	FRI	SAT

This month I accomplished: _____
_____
_____

Notes: _____
_____
_____
_____

October | Extra Credit

I will give my child a DHA supplement every day, preferably at breakfast.

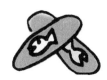

SUN	MON	TUE	WED	THU	FRI	SAT

This month I accomplished: _____

_____

_____

Notes: _____

_____

_____

_____

November | Goal

I will add ½ cup of fruits or vegetables each week until my child meets the recommended intake (at least 3 to 5 cups daily based on age).

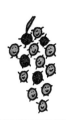

SUN	MON	TUE	WED	THU	FRI	SAT

This month I accomplished: _____

_____

_____

Notes: _____

_____

_____

_____

November | Extra Credit

I will serve a fruit or veggie in each color group (purple, red, orange-yellow, green and white) at least three days per week.

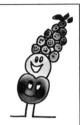

SUN	MON	TUE	WED	THU	FRI	SAT

This month I accomplished: _____

_____

_____

Notes: _____

_____

_____

_____

December | Goal

I will enforce a regular bedtime hour to help my child get enough memory-enhancing REM sleep at least five times per week.

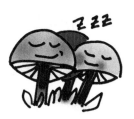

SUN	MON	TUE	WED	THU	FRI	SAT

This month I accomplished: _____

_____

_____

Notes: _____

_____

_____

_____

December | Extra Credit

I will sprinkle an antioxidant-rich spice on my child's food each day or include a daily serving of a "Star Power" food (see page 83).

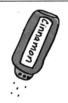

SUN	MON	TUE	WED	THU	FRI	SAT

This month I accomplished: _____

_____

_____

Notes: _____

_____

_____

January | Goal

I will have my child help out with the planning and making of school lunches at least once a week.

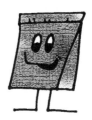

SUN	MON	TUE	WED	THU	FRI	SAT

This month I accomplished: _____

_____

_____

Notes: _____

_____

_____

January | Extra Credit

I will include a joke, riddle, brainteaser or other fun pick in my child's lunch box at least twice a week.

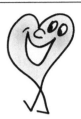

SUN	MON	TUE	WED	THU	FRI	SAT

This month I accomplished: _____

_____

_____

Notes: _____

_____

_____

February | Goal

I will have my child help create one complete meal for the family this month (grocery shopping, cooking and setting the table).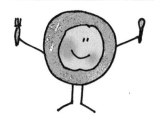

SUN	MON	TUE	WED	THU	FRI	SAT

This month I accomplished: _____

_____

_____

Notes: _____

_____

_____

February | Extra Credit

I will play Rate Your Plate with my child at three meals per week (and earn at least 5 points per session).

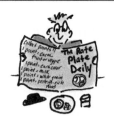

SUN	MON	TUE	WED	THU	FRI	SAT

This month I accomplished: _____

_____

_____

Notes: _____

_____

_____

March | Goal

I will add 5 minutes of jumping, running or other fun activities until my child is active at least 60 minutes every day. (Take it one step at a time—listen to your child—and make sure it's fun!)

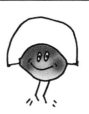

SUN	MON	TUE	WED	THU	FRI	SAT

This month I accomplished: _____

_____

_____

Notes: _____

_____

_____

March | Extra Credit

I will help my child limit TV to no more than 2 hours per day.

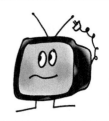

SUN	MON	TUE	WED	THU	FRI	SAT

This month I accomplished: _____

_____

_____

Notes: _____

_____

_____

April | Goal

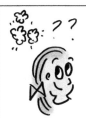 I will help my child brainstorm a healthier substitute to one of his or her frequent junk food choices this month.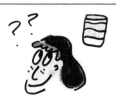

SUN	MON	TUE	WED	THU	FRI	SAT

This month I accomplished: _____

_____

_____

Notes: _____

_____

_____

April | Extra Credit

I will help my child learn his or her recommended "empty-calorie" limit.

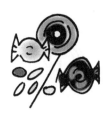

SUN	MON	TUE	WED	THU	FRI	SAT

This month I accomplished: _____

_____

_____

Notes: _____

_____

_____

May | Goal

I will serve at least one new fruit, vegetable or whole grain food each week.

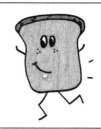

SUN	MON	TUE	WED	THU	FRI	SAT

This month I accomplished: _____

_____

_____

Notes: _____

_____

_____

May | Extra Credit

I will start a "square foot" garden.

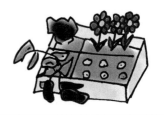

SUN	MON	TUE	WED	THU	FRI	SAT

This month I accomplished: _____

_____

_____

Notes: _____

_____

_____

June | Goal

I will have my child track urine color and drink more fluid if the color resembles that of apple juice.

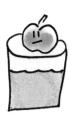

SUN	MON	TUE	WED	THU	FRI	SAT

This month I accomplished: _____

_____

_____

Notes: _____

_____

_____

June | Extra Credit

I will make a summer "To Do" list with my family of activities that stimulate both mind and body.

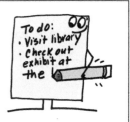

SUN	MON	TUE	WED	THU	FRI	SAT

This month I accomplished: _____
_____
_____

Notes: _____
_____
_____

July | Goal

I will read the Nutrition Facts on packaged foods to choose brands with zero grams of trans fats.

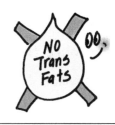

SUN	MON	TUE	WED	THU	FRI	SAT

This month I accomplished: _____

_____

_____

Notes: _____

_____

_____

July | Extra Credit

I will serve portions of packaged foods that are no more than the serving size listed on the Nutrition Facts panel.

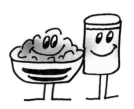

SUN	MON	TUE	WED	THU	FRI	SAT

This month I accomplished: _____

_____

_____

Notes: _____

_____

_____

August | Goal

At least two weeks before school starts, I will establish a homework space based on the "Better Homework" tips.

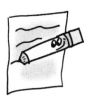

SUN	MON	TUE	WED	THU	FRI	SAT

This month I accomplished: _____

_____

_____

Notes: _____

_____

_____

August | Extra Credit

At least two weeks before school starts, I will buy a backpack based on the "Backpack Know-How" tips.

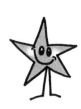

SUN	MON	TUE	WED	THU	FRI	SAT

This month I accomplished: _____

_____

_____

Notes: _____

_____

_____

Month:_____ | Goal

I will _____

_____

_____

SUN	MON	TUE	WED	THU	FRI	SAT

This month I accomplished: _____

_____

_____

Notes: _____

_____

_____

Month:_____ | Goal

I will _____

_____

_____

SUN	MON	TUE	WED	THU	FRI	SAT

This month I accomplished: _____

_____

_____

Notes: _____

_____

_____

Month:_____ | Goal

I will _____

_____

_____

SUN	MON	TUE	WED	THU	FRI	SAT

This month I accomplished: _____

_____

_____

Notes: _____

_____

_____

Month:_____ | Goal

I will _____

_____

_____

SUN	MON	TUE	WED	THU	FRI	SAT

This month I accomplished: _____

_____

_____

Notes: _____

_____

_____

Month:_____ | Goal

I will _____

_____

_____

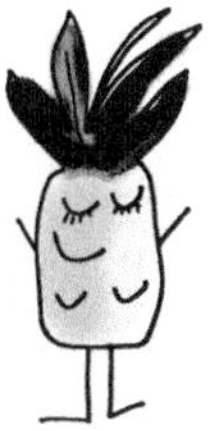

SUN	MON	TUE	WED	THU	FRI	SAT

This month I accomplished: _____

_____

_____

Notes: _____

_____

_____

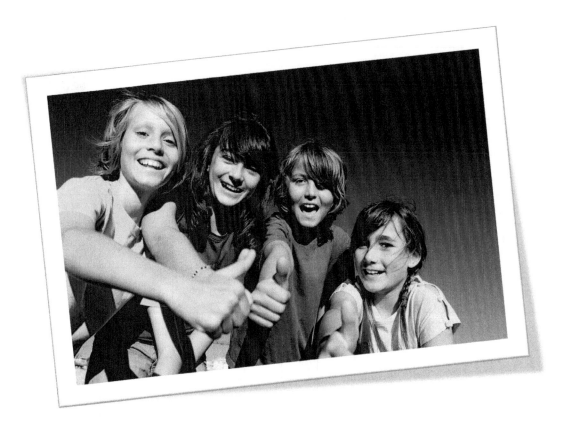

We can all agree that in the wealthiest nation on Earth, all children should have the basic nutrition they need to learn and grow and to pursue their dreams, because in the end, nothing is more important than the health and well-being of our children. Nothing.
– Michelle Obama

Chapter 15

Tables, Tips & More

In this chapter, you'll find a wide variety of at-a-glance resources to help you fuel your child's growing body and active brain. You'll find guidelines for your child's intake of daily calories—including empty calories—to help achieve and maintain a healthy body weight. You'll also find the recommended intake of vitamins, minerals and macronutrients—protein, fat, carbohydrate and fiber—to fuel your child's day. And, to translate daily calories into foods to serve your child, you'll find the recommended daily portions for each food group.

We know kids don't eat nutrition; they eat enticing foods that taste great. To inspire you to serve up healthy options, you'll find substitution tips to pack more nutrition into your favorite recipes without compromising flavor, what foods to stock in your fridge, freezer and pantry, and what tools to keep on hand to make your kitchen time even more enjoyable. Here's a list of the resources you'll find in this chapter:

- Recipe Makeover Tips & Tricks
- Stocking Your Fridge, Freezer & Pantry
- Choosing Kitchen Utensils & Tools

- Recommended Daily Intake: Calories
- Recommended Daily "Empty" Calorie Limit
- Sample Serving Sizes for Each Food Group
- Recommended Daily Intake: Food Groups
- Recommended Daily Intake: Vitamins
- Recommended Daily Intake: Minerals
- Recommended Daily Intake: Macronutrients

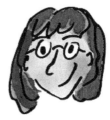

Did You Know?

Organically grown fruits and vegetables often contain higher amounts of vitamin C and antioxidant flavonoids compared with conventionally grown varieties. Organic produce also tends to be more flavorful—a key selling point to entice your kids to get their daily quota.

Recipe Makeover Tips & Tricks

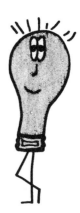

With a few minor adjustments, you can maximize the health benefits of your favorite recipes. The key is to focus on cutting the fat and sugar and boosting the fiber in a way that keeps the flavor impact high. Here are our best kitchen-tested and kid-approved makeover secrets to transform your favorite recipes into more nutrient-packed fuel for your child's active brain without compromising flavor.

Tips to Cut Fat

- **Reach for applesauce.** In recipes for most quick breads, muffin or other baked goods, you can replace up to half of the butter, oil or shortening with applesauce or dried plum (prune) puree without dramatically affecting texture.

- **Skip the cream.** Transform creamy sauces into lower fat alternatives by replacing cream with evaporated skim milk, light cream or non-fat half-and-half. Add a little flour as a thickening agent to help maintain a smooth consistency.

- **Use non-stick pans or vegetable oil sprays.** This simply change will dramatically reduce the amount of fat needed for cooking.

- **Add a rack when roasting.** Placing poultry or meat on a rack will allow the excess fat to drip off.

- **Switch to lower fat dairy products.** Substituting low-fat or non-fat dairy products for whole fat varieties in your recipes will reduce the fat without altering flavor.

- **Cook soups and gravies and refrigerate overnight**. This allows enough time for excess fat to congeal on the top for easy skimming.

- **Substitute with plain yogurt.** Plain yogurt is an ideal substitute for recipes that call for sour cream or mayonnaise.

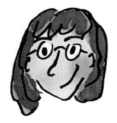

Did You Know?

Dietary fiber is the term used to describe material from plant cells that the body's enzymes can't digest. You won't find it in animal-based foods — not even the toughest steaks.

Based on scientific research, the best sources of fiber include the following:

- Unrefined whole grain breads and cereals
- Legumes such as pinto and kidney beans
- Vegetables, especially peas, broccoli, spinach, tomatoes, potatoes, carrots, corn and green peppers
- Fresh fruits with skins or seeds such as apples, apricots, pears, plums and berries

Tips to Cut Sugar

- **Reduce sugar gradually in a recipe.** Most recipes allow for cutting the amount of refined sugar by about one-fourth—and in some cases up to one-third—without affecting taste or texture.

- **Substitute apple juice concentrate for sugar in baked goods.** This is our go-to staple to cut the sugar in recipes. Here's a good rule-of-thumb: For every one cup of sugar, substitute ¾ cup apple juice concentrate while decreasing the amount of liquid in the recipe by three tablespoons.

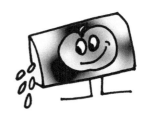

- **Serve sweet foods warm.** Heat enhances the perception of sweetness, helping you to retain the flavor while cutting the sugar.

Tips to Boost Fiber

- **Gradually add more fiber to your child's diet.** This allows the digestive tract to adjust. Adding more dietary fiber too quickly may lead to digestive upset and stomach ache.

- **Choose carbohydrates in their natural fibrous coatings.** For example, brown rice instead of white rice or whole grain crackers, breads and cereals instead of their white counterparts. In many recipes, you can replace up to half of the white flour with a whole grain flour.

- **Serve more vegetables and fruits with edible skins and seeds**. These plant parts are good sources of dietary fiber. Simply wash and serve.

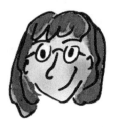

Did You Know?

Apples, bananas, grapes, strawberries and oranges top the list of fruit favorites for kids, 6 to 12 years old. The top veggies are corn, green beans, carrots and peas.

Stocking Your Fridge, Freezer & Pantry

Stocking your kitchen with healthy foods is one of the easiest ways to ensure your child has nutrient-rich choices at the ready when hunger strikes. Read on for a list of staples for your refrigerator, freezer and pantry along with kid-friendly serving suggestions that are sure to please.

Foods for Your Refrigerator

- **Cottage cheese (non-fat or low-fat).** Serve with fruit or in salads, or toss with cooked pasta and vegetables with a sprinkle of parmesan cheese.

- **Cheese.** Serve sliced on whole wheat crackers, melted over a whole grain bagel or grated in a fresh salad.

- **Eggs.** Serve poached, scrambled or boiled, and consider buying DHA-enriched eggs for a brain boost.

- **Flax (milled).** Sprinkle on cereal and add in recipes for extra omega-3 protection.

- **Milk (non-fat or low-fat).** Pour over cereals, blend into smoothies or enjoy as a nutritious beverage all by itself.

- **Pre-cut veggies and fruit.** Pre-cut and ready to serve makes for a great time saver when hunger strikes.

- **Yogurt (non-fat or low-fat, plain or flavored).** Mix with fresh fruit for a yogurt parfait or use a plain variety to replace mayonnaise in salad dressings or sour cream on a baked potato.

Foods for Your Freezer

- **Bread products.** Whole wheat bread and rolls, English muffins and pita bread are kid-friendly and make for fast and healthy options when toasted and topped with low-fat cheese, peanut butter, no-added-sugar jams or apple butter.

- **Frozen fruit pieces (with no added sugar).** Use for a quick dessert idea or blend with non-fat or low-fat milk or yogurt for a thick shake.

- **Frozen vegetables (no added cream or butter).** Serve as a side dish, add to pasta or top a baked potato sprinkled with low-fat cheese.

- **Frozen fish (such as salmon), chicken or other lean meats.** Stir fry with vegetables, serve on top of a salad or mix with pasta.

- **Frozen ground turkey.** This versatile staple is great for turkey burgers and in meat loaf, spaghetti sauce and taco filling.

- **Frozen burgers (turkey, veggie or lean meat).** Ideal for a quick meal when you're in pinch.

- **Frozen fresh herbs (washed).** Toss into a freezer bag, label and date for ready access.

Foods for Your Pantry

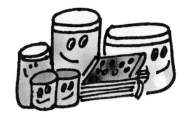

- **Canned tomato products (diced, sauce or paste).** Ideal to add to homemade soups or pasta sauce. Tomato sauce or paste makes an easy topping for a toasted English muffin: simply spread, add grated low-fat cheese and broil.

- **Canned tuna, salmon and beans such as pinto, garbanzo and kidney.** Drain, rinse and add to salads, soups and stews.

- **Flour.** Keep this recipe staple at the ready, but store whole wheat in the refrigerator.

- **Grains (whole).** Consider amaranth, brown rice, buckwheat, couscous, kamut, kasha, pasta, quinoa, triticale berries, rye berries, spelt (farro) or wheat berries. Ideal for side dishes, in casseroles or as a topping for stir-fried vegetables.

- **Herbs (assorted) and other flavor enhancers.** Herbs, spices, salt-free seasonings, grated parmesan cheese, vanilla and other extracts are great flavor enhancers to spice up recipes and add variety to your child's diet.

- **Oat bran and oats (rolled or steel-cut).** Serve as breakfast cereal or use in baking.

- **Peanut butter (old-fashioned).** For easier stirring, store the sealed jar upside down until ready to open to allow the natural oils to move throughout jar. Refrigerate after opening.

- **Popcorn.** Air-popped as a snack.

- **Potatoes, yams or sweet potatoes.** For an easy, filling meal, bake or microwave and top with vegetables and a protein source. Add to soups and salads or enjoy as leftovers for breakfast. Be sure to store in a cool, dry place.

- **Sugar**. Although you'll likely be using less of this staple in your recipes or sprinkled on foods, it's good to keep some on hand.

- **Unsweetened applesauce, no-sugar-added jams or apple butter.** An ideal substitute for butter as a spread for toast or topping for pancakes.

- **Vegetable oil (such as canola and olive) and vinegar.** For salad dressings and in cooking.

- **Whole wheat crackers.** A quick and nutritious snack.

Extras

- **Multivitamin**. A high-quality children's complete multivitamin/mineral supplement—with iron and omega-3 DHA. This daily habit helps fill potential nutrient gaps between your child's typical diet and what their active brain needs.

Choosing Kitchen Utensils & Tools

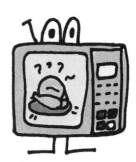

Good kitchen tools can make the difference between having fun in the kitchen or sweating away in misery. Choose high-quality items that will last. Read on for a list of need-to-have kitchen utensils and other tools—as well as a few nice-to-have choices—and tips on features to look for to make your time in the kitchen more enjoyable.

Appliances

- **Blender.** Look for sturdy blades, a rubber base, a glass pitcher and at least one horsepower, especially if smoothies are part of your regular routine.

- **Hand-held beater.** Choose a brand with a case for easy storage of all the parts and pieces that tend to wander.

- **Microwave oven.** Look for an energy-efficient model with a turntable plate, easy-to-read controls, a straight-forward setting sequence and a bright interior light.

  Slow Cooker. Look for a removable pot for easy cleaning, a sturdy base and a timer to prevent overcooking. A 6-quart size is perfect for preparing meals for up to six people.

Bakeware

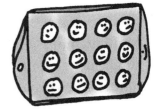

- **Baking pans (non-stick).** Most recipes call for an 8- or 9-inch square pan or a 9x12-inch rectangular pan.

- **Cookie sheets (non-stick).** Heavy-gauge aluminum with low or no sides, a dull finish and a lighter color (to help reduce burning).

- **Loaf pan (non-stick).** Most recipes for banana, zucchini or other kid-friendly quick breads require a 9x5-inch loaf pan.

- **Muffin tins (non-stick).** Consider a tin designed for mini muffins for kid-friendly portions.

- **Pie pan (non-stick).** Consider a pan with an 8- or 9-inch diameter.

Pots and Pans

- **Mixing bowls.** Stainless steel of various sizes that fit within each other for easy storage.

- **Pots.** Stainless steel with covers; most cooks use 1½-quart and 3-quart pots or a 4-quart Dutch oven. For serious homemade soups, consider a 12-quart stock pot.

- **Skillets.** Look for stainless steel, iron or non-stick. Consider one small (7-inch diameter) and one large (12-inch diameter) skillet, which would meet most food prep needs.

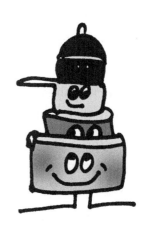

Gadgets

- **Bottle opener.** Choose a sturdy, old-fashioned style with two ends: one blunt for bottles; the other pointed for cans.

- **Can opener.** Choose a model that cuts around the outside of the can, rather than the lid. The result is a smooth edge and a lid that won't fall into the food.

- **Cheese slicer.** Choose a brand with a sturdy handle. Consider having two—a cheese plane for hard cheese and a cheese knife for softer varieties.

- **Cookie cutters.** Choose kid-friendly shapes without intricate designs.

- **Cooking thermometer.** Choose an instant, easy-to-read, shatter-proof thermometer with a case.

- **Cutting board.** Wood or plastic—experts have yet to agree which is more sanitary. Choose the biggest board that your space allows. A smaller one for little jobs may also be helpful.

- **Grater.** Best to get at least two: a flat one and a boxed one with different size holes. Plastic graters are safer for children.

- **Ice cube trays.** Choose trays with lids to freeze fruit or vegetable purees for smoothies or soup stocks, respectively.

- **Kitchen knives.** Consider a countertop set that includes a chef's knife, paring knife and serrated slicing knife.

- **Kitchen shears.** Keep in the kitchen and use only with food in mind.

- **Lettuce spinner.** Choose a brand with a plunger—rather than a spinner—feature for wash and spin dry action that's easy on the wrists.

- **Measuring cups.** Choose a brand with a one-piece design and non-collapsible plastic that won't fall apart when full or break if dropped.

- **Measuring spoons.** Choose an oval—rather than round—shape that's easier to fit into tight spice jars.

- **Peeler.** Choose one that can double as an apple corer.

- **Spatulas.** Consider having a metal one to handle delicate items such as cookies and a rubber one for heavier items such as burgers.

- **Timer.** Choose a digital model with a multiple timekeeping function to track more than one food—a roast in the oven, potatoes on the stove and rising dough on the counter.

- **Tongs.** Look for fluid movement and not-too-tight spring tension. Examine the tips and make sure they are no more than 6 inches apart to make them less tiresome to hold.

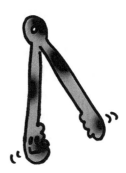

- **Utensils.** Look for dishwasher safe utensils to save time and ensure cleanliness.

- **Wooden spoons.** Choose ones with comfortable handles.

Nice-to-Have Supplies

- **Dishware (durable and chip-resistant).** From table to storage, durable, chip-resistant dishware is an ideal choice for families with young school-aged children. Choosing a pattern with a solid color allows you to dress it up with cheerful napkins.

- **Canisters.** Splurge on a brand with an air-lock feature for longer shelf-life of grains and other items.

- **Food clips.** Consider using file clips, which are typically a less expensive option.

- **Pot holders.** Consider buying a few to keep handy or oven gloves for added protection.

- **Vegetable brush.** Choose a sturdy model that is easy to grip firmly.

- **Plastic storage bags.** Plastic freezer bags allow removal of air and ease of labeling.

- **Permanent marker.** Keep a permanent marker in a kitchen drawer for handy labeling of plastic bags with leftovers.

Recommended Daily Intake: Calories

The recommended daily calorie intake for your child depends on many factors such as activity level, age, height and weight. Counting calories is generally unnecessary, but knowing a ballpark number can help you plan a healthy diet. The chart below provides an estimate of the recommended daily calorie intake for girls and boys, age 4 to 13 years.

Recommended Daily Calorie Intake for Girls and Boys		
	Sedentary*	**Physically Active****
Girls		
4 to 8 years old	1,200 calories	1,400 to 1,800 calories
9 to 13 years old	1,600 calories	1,600 to 2,200 calories
Boys		
4 to 8 years old	1,400 calories	1,400 to 2,000 calories
9 to 13 years old	1,800 calories	1,800 to 2,600 calories
*Less than 30 minutes of moderate physical activity on most days. **At least 30 minutes (lower calorie level) to at least 60 minutes (higher calorie level) of moderate physical activity on most days. Adapted from: www.choosemyplate.gov.		

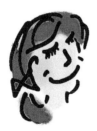

Recommended Daily "Empty Calorie" Limit

No food is forbidden, but every one counts. The chart below provides a recommended limit for "empty calorie" foods for girls and boys, age 4 to 13 years. These foods are typically high in added fat or sugar, but devoid of any nutritional value. Nonetheless, these foods won't derail an otherwise healthy diet when they make up no more than 10 percent of the total daily calorie intake.

Recommended "Empty Calorie" Limit for Girls and Boys		
	Sedentary*	**Physically Active****
Girls		
4 to 8 years old	no more than 120 calories	no more than 140 to 180 calories
9 to 13 years old	no more than 160 calories	no more than 160 to 220 calories
Boys		
4 to 8 years old	no more than 140 calories	no more than 140 to 200 calories
9 to 13 years old	no more than 180 calories	no more than 180 to 260 calories

*Less than 30 minutes of moderate physical activity on most days.
**At least 30 minutes (lower calorie level) to at least 60 minutes (higher calorie level) of moderate physical activity on most days.
Adapted from: www.choosemyplate.gov.

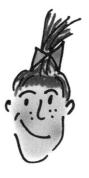
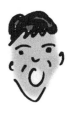

Sample Serving Sizes for Each Food Group

Fruit

One serving equals:

- 1 cup fruit or fruit juice
- ½ cup dried fruit

Protein and Legumes

One serving equals:

- 1 ounce meat, poultry or fish
- ¼ cup cooked dry beans
- 1 egg
- ½ ounce nuts

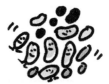

Vegetables

One serving equals:

- 1 cup raw or cooked
- 2 cups leafy greens
- 1 cup veggie juice

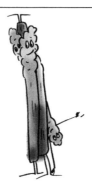

Grains

One serving equals:

- ½ cup cooked cereal, rice or pasta
- 1 slice bread
- 1 cup dry cereal
- ½ muffin
- 1 mini bagel

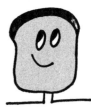

Dairy

One serving equals:

- 1 cup milk
- 1 cup yogurt
- 1½ ounce cheese

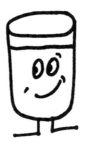

Fat

One serving equals:

- 1 teaspoon oil
- 1 teaspoon butter (1 pat)

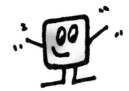

Adapted from: www.choosemyplate.gov/food-groups/.

Recommended Daily Intake: Food Groups

The recommended daily food intake for your child is listed below by food group. You'll want to know how closely your child's intake matches the recommended intake for their age and gender. To spot check, keep a one-day food record. Here's how: Tomorrow, write down all the foods and beverages your child eats, including the amounts. Remember to ask about foods eaten while at school and away from home. Compare the one-day food record to the recommended intakes listed in the chart below.

Recommended Daily Intake by Food Group for Girls and Boys*			
	4 to 8 years old	**9 to 13 years old**	
Food Group	**Girls and Boys**	**Girls**	**Boys**
Fruit	1 to 1½ servings	1½ servings	1½ servings
Vegetables	1½ servings	2 servings	2½ servings
Grains	5 servings	5 servings	6 servings
Protein and Legumes	4 servings	5 servings	5 servings
Dairy	2 servings	3 servings	3 servings
Fat	4 servings	5 servings	5 servings

* For sedentary children who get less than 30 minutes of moderate physical activity per day, beyond normal daily activities. Physically active children may require more to meet their calorie needs. Adapted from: www.choosemyplate.gov/food-groups/.

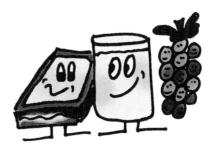

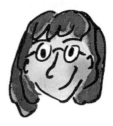

Did You Know?

Fruits and vegetables are a treasure trove of nutrients and beneficial phytochemicals that deliver antioxidant protection.

Young children, 4 to 8 years, should consume at least 2½ servings of fruits and vegetables in a variety of colors every day, while older children, 9 to 13 years, should aim for a daily intake of at least 3½ servings.

Recommended Daily Intake: Vitamins

Recommended Daily Intake for Girls and Boys: Vitamins		
Vitamin	**4 to 8 years**	**9 to 13 years**
Vitamin A	400 micrograms	600 micrograms
Vitamin C	25 milligrams	45 milligrams
Vitamin D	5 micrograms	5 micrograms
Vitamin E	7 milligrams	11 milligrams
Vitamin K	55 micrograms	60 micrograms
Thiamin (Vitamin B1)	0.6 milligrams	0.9 milligrams
Riboflavin (Vitamin B2)	0.6 milligrams	0.9 milligrams
Niacin	8 milligrams	12 milligrams
Vitamin B6	0.6 milligrams	1 milligram
Folate	200 micrograms	300 micrograms
Vitamin B12	1.2 micrograms	1.8 micrograms
Pantothenic Acid	3 milligrams	4 milligrams
Biotin	12 micrograms	20 micrograms
Choline	250 milligrams	375 milligrams
Source: Institute of Medicine. *DRI Reference Intakes: The Essential Guide to Nutrient Requirements.* Washington, DC: The National Academies Press; 2006.		

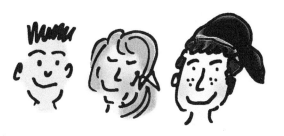

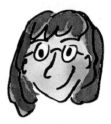

Did You Know?

Variety in your child's diet is important to help ensure an adequate amount of all the essential nutrients—over 35 vitamins, minerals and macronutrients—as well as emerging nutrients such as health-promoting phytochemicals.

One of the easiest ways to boost variety is to tap into your child's quest for flavorful foods. The bonus: Trying new food taste sensations can be a fun adventure.

Recommended Daily Intake: Minerals

Recommended Daily Intake for Girls and Boys: Minerals		
Mineral	**4 to 8 years**	**9 to 13 years**
Calcium	800 milligrams	1300 milligrams
Chromium	15 micrograms	21 micrograms (girls)
		25 micrograms (boys)
Copper	440 micrograms	700 micrograms
Fluoride	1 milligram	2 milligrams
Iodine	90 micrograms	120 micrograms
Iron	10 milligrams	8 milligrams
Magnesium	130 milligrams	240 milligrams
Manganese	1.5 milligrams	1.6 milligrams (girls)
		1.9 milligrams (boys)
Molybdenum	22 micrograms	34 micrograms
Phosphorus	500 milligrams	1250 milligrams
Selenium	30 micrograms	40 micrograms
Zinc	5 milligrams	8 milligrams
Potassium	3.8 grams	4.5 grams
Sodium	1.2 grams	1.5 grams
Chloride	1.9 grams	2.3 grams
Source: Institute of Medicine. *DRI Reference Intakes: The Essential Guide to Nutrient Requirements*. Washington, DC: The National Academies Press; 2006.		

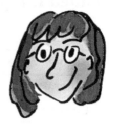

Did You Know?

Every system in your child's body requires water. An adequate intake is essential to aid digestion, bring nutrients and oxygen to the cells, remove waste products and maintain normal metabolism.

While foods contribute some water to your child's total daily intake, most of it comes from drinking water and other beverages. So, encourage your child to drink up. Here's the breakdown:

	Total Water	From Beverages	From Food
Girls			
4 to 8 years old	7 cups	5 cups	2 cups
9 to 13 years old	9 cups	7 cups	2 cups
Boys			
4 to 8 years old	7 cups	5 cups	2 cups
9 to 13 years old	10 cups	8 cups	2 cups

Source: Institute of Medicine. *DRI Reference Intakes: The Essential Guide to Nutrient Requirements.* Washington, DC: The National Academies Press; 2006.

Recommended Daily Intake: Macronutrients

Recommended Daily Intake for Girls and Boys: Macronutrients		
Macronutrient	**4 to 8 years**	**9 to 13 years**
Total Water*	7 cups	9 cups (girls)
		10 cups (boys)
Carbohydrates	130 grams	130 grams
Protein	19 grams	34 grams
Fat	Not Determined	Not Determined
Linoleic Acid (Omega-6 Fat)	10 grams	10 grams (girls)
		12 grams (boys)
Linolenic Acid (Omega-3 Fat)	0.9 grams	1.0 gram (girls)
		1.2 grams (boys)
Fiber	25 grams	26 grams (girls)
		31 grams (boys)

*Includes water contained in food, beverages and drinking water.
Source: Institute of Medicine. *DRI Reference Intakes: The Essential Guide to Nutrient Requirements.* Washington, DC: The National Academies Press; 2006.

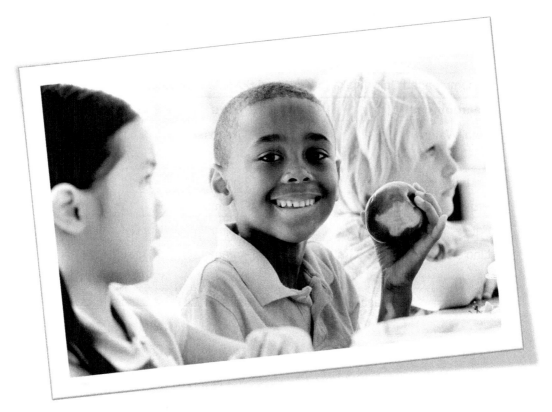

Children are like wet cement.
Whatever falls on them makes an impression.
— Dr. Haim Ginott

Chapter 16

Glossary

Acetylcholine – An important chemical messenger in the brain for cell-to-cell communication involved in learning, memory and other functions.

Active child - A child who gets at least 30 to 60 minutes of moderate physical activity on most days.

Alpha-linolenic acid (ALA) – An essential omega-3 fatty acid.

Amino acid - A protein building block.

Anthocyanins – Red, purple and blue plant pigments with strong antioxidant properties.

Antioxidants – Protective nutrients such as vitamins C and E and numerous naturally occurring plant compounds. In the body, antioxidants help protect against harmful free radicals.

Bioflavanoids – Antioxidant compounds found as pigments in many fruits and vegetables.

Biotin – A B vitamin involved in the metabolism of carbohydrates and the synthesis of fats and proteins.

Body mass index (BMI) – An estimate of body fat and predictor of overall health.

Brain-derived neurotropic factor (BDNF) – A chemical in the brain that is responsible for the development of new brain tissue.

Caffeine – A compound found in foods, beverages and over-the-counter drugs designed to fight fatigue. It has a stimulating effect that can last for several hours and a diuretic effect (increases the body's ability to expel water) that can lead to dehydration.

Calcium – A mineral that is essential in the formation of strong bones and teeth. It also stimulates blood clotting after injury and is required for normal muscle and nerve activity. Adequate calcium intake may reduce the risk of osteoporosis later in life.

Calorie – A unit of measure used to express the energy in foods.

Carbohydrate – The principle source of energy in the diet (providing 4 calories per gram). The two main types are simple carbohydrates (simple sugars) and complex carbohydrates (starch and fiber).

Carotenoids – Plant pigments with antioxidant properties including beta-carotene, lutein, alpha-carotene and lycopene.

Choline – A chemical cousin to the B vitamin family; serves as a building block for phosphatidylcholine.

Chromium – A trace mineral that is essential for the normal metabolism of glucose. It also influences carbohydrate, fat and protein metabolism. Refining food leads to appreciable losses of chromium.

Complex carbohydrate – A compound containing long chains of simple sugars that provides a sustained increase in energy.

Copper – A trace mineral involved in iron metabolism, nervous system functioning, bone health and the synthesis of proteins. It is an essential component of an antioxidant enzyme and also plays a role in the pigmentation of skin, hair and eyes.

Docosahexaenoic acid (DHA) – An essential omega-3 fatty acid.

Eicosapentaenoic acid (EPA) – An essential omega-3 fatty acid.

Enzyme – A compound produced by cells to help activate or speed up biochemical reactions.

Fat – An essential nutrient that provides concentrated energy (9 calories per gram), contributes to the taste of food, acts as a carrier of fat-soluble vitamins and supplies essential fatty acids.

Fiber – A type of complex carbohydrate that exhibits various degrees of resistance to human digestion. It is found only in foods of plant origin.

Flavonoids – Powerful antioxidants found in plants that protect against oxidative damage caused by harmful free radicals.

Folic acid – Also known as folate, this B vitamin works hand in hand with vitamin B12. It is essential to regulate and maintain overall cellular health, healthy cell division and the formation of new cells, including red blood cells.

Food neophobia – A fear of new foods.

Free radicals – Unstable and highly reactive compounds that are formed during normal metabolism, but dramatically increase with exposure to sun, air pollution, smoking and other damaging environmental factors as well as from intense exercise. With an adequate intake of antioxidants, the body can neutralize free radicals before they can harm cells and tissues.

Glycemic Index (GI) – A system of ranking foods based on how they affect blood glucose levels immediately after being consumed.

Glycogen – The main storage form of carbohydrates in the body.

Indoles – A type of phytonutrient and enzyme inducer derived from cruciferous vegetables such as broccoli, cauliflower and cabbage.

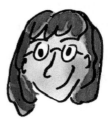

Did You Know?

Sunflower seeds may help boost memory. Emerging research in laboratory animals suggests that eating foods with oleic acid—a fatty acid found in sunflower seeds—may help improve your child's ability to remember.

Iodine – As part of the thyroid hormone, this mineral helps regulate growth, development and energy metabolism. Seafood, such as shellfish, fish and seaweed, are the best sources of iodine.

Iron – A trace mineral that is an essential part of hemoglobin, a compound which carries oxygen in the blood. Iron is also involved in energy metabolism. Iron deficiency anemia is a common health problem in children.

Lutein – A carotenoid that is found in fruits and veggies and functions as an antioxidant.

Lycopene – A carotenoid that gives fruits and veggies their red and pink colors. Lycopene has been shown to provide antioxidant activity, and a diet rich in lycopene has been associated with prostate and heart health.

Macronutrient – A nutrient that is required in large (gram) amounts; includes carbohydrate, fat, protein, fiber and water.

Magnesium – A mineral required for normal muscle (including heart muscle) and nerve activity. It is involved in the metabolism of ATP, the cellular energy compound, and DNA, the genetic material.

Manganese – A trace mineral that is necessary for the normal development of skeletal and connective tissues. It is involved in fatty acid synthesis and carbohydrate metabolism. Low intakes of manganese may lead to porous bone.

Memory consolidation – A type of cognitive process that converts new information into a lasting memory.

Micronutrient – A nutrient, including vitamins and some minerals, that is required by the body in small (milligram or microgram) amounts.

Mineral – An indestructible element that cannot be destroyed by heat, acid or air. Unlike a vitamin, a mineral is not produced by a living organism. A mineral that is required for human health is known as an "essential mineral."

Molybdenum – A trace mineral that is an essential part of several enzymes in the body. It may be involved in the metabolism of the hormone glucocorticoid.

Neurotoxin – A substance that causes damage to nerves or nerve tissue.

Neurotransmitter – A chemical, released from a nerve cell, that transmits an impulse from the nerve cell to another nerve cell, muscle, organ or other tissue.

Nerve growth factors – A naturally occurring molecule in the body that stimulates the growth and differentiation of the sympathetic and certain sensory nerves.

Niacin (Vitamin B3) – A B vitamin that is essential for the release of energy from carbohydrates, fats and proteins. It helps maintain healthy skin and plays a role in blood sugar control.

Norepinephrine – An important neurotransmitter that helps sustain attention and the ability to concentrate.

Omega-3-fatty acids – A class of fatty acids that includes DHA, the essential fatty acid that supports optimal health, especially heart, brain and eye health. An adequate dietary intake of fatty acids in this class helps counterbalance a high dietary intake of omega-6 fatty acids.

ORAC (Oxygen Radical Absorbance Capacity) – A type of laboratory test that researchers use to measure the antioxidant capacity of a food.

Organic – Chemically, a substance containing carbon in the molecule. The U.S. Department of Agriculture (USDA) also permits the use of the term on foods that meet certain standards. For plant-based foods, the requirement is from plants grown without the use of synthetic pesticides, fungicides or inorganic fertilizers. For animal-based foods, the requirement is from animals raised on organic feed that is free of any parts of slaughtered animals, allowed outside and not given antibiotics or growth hormones.

Oxidative stress – A condition that occurs when the production of free radicals exceeds the body's normal ability to neutralize and eliminate them. This condition may occur with excessive exposure to sun, air pollution, smoking and other damaging environmental factors as well as from intense exercise.

Oxygen Radical Absorbance Capacity – see ORAC.

Pantothenic Acid (Vitamin B5) – A B vitamin that helps release energy from foods and is a key component of fat metabolism. A significant loss of this vitamin occurs when food is processed.

Phosphatidylcholine – Also known as lecithin; a fat-like compound important for the structural integrity of cell membranes and chemical signaling between cells.

Phosphorous – An essential mineral that forms bones and teeth and regulates energy release from foods. It is a component of the body's major energy source, ATP, and the genetic material, DNA.

Phytonutrients – A naturally occurring plant compound, many of which have health-protecting properties.

Protein – An organic compound made up of amino acids. Proteins are needed for growth, maintenance and repair of tissue. They are vital for the regulation of body processes, and are especially important during periods of growth. Protein provides 4 calories per gram.

Quercetin – An antioxidant in the flavonoid family that occurs naturally in foods such as apples, red grapes and tea.

Riboflavin (Vitamin B2) – A B vitamin that assists in production of energy from foods and the formation of red blood cells. It is involved in numerous metabolic reactions.

Saturated fat – A type of fat that is generally solid at room temperature and commonly found in meats and foods of animal origin.

Sedentary child – A child who gets less than 30 minutes of moderate physical activity on most days.

Selenium – An essential trace mineral that acts as an antioxidant. Recent discoveries indicate that selenium is also important in the metabolism of thyroid hormones.

Serotonin – An important neurotransmitter that helps sustain attention and the ability to concentrate.

Simple carbohydrate – A compound containing only one or two simple sugars that provides quick energy.

Starch – A type of complex carbohydrate consisting of long chains of simple sugars that is digestible by humans. It is found only in foods of plant origin.

Thiamin (Vitamin B1) – A B vitamin that assists in carbohydrate metabolism and energy production. It is required for normal nerve function and may play a role in brain function.

Unsaturated fat – A type of fat that is generally fluid at room temperature (e.g., cooking oil) and generally derived from plants. When hydrogen atoms are added to make them firmer, they are called "partially hydrogenated vegetable oils."

Vitamin – A compound, essential for life, that is produced by living organisms. Vitamins are free of calories and required by the body in only small (milligram or microgram) amounts.

Vitamin A – An essential vitamin required for vision, growth and bone development. It plays a role in the proper functioning of most organs in the body and the body's natural immune defense, including helping to maintain healthy skin and mucous membranes.

Vitamin B6 (Pyridoxine) – A B vitamin that is essential for protein metabolism, nervous system and immune system function and plays a role in the synthesis of hormones and red blood cells.

Vitamin B12 (Cobalamin) – A B vitamin that is essential for normal growth and the production of red blood cells. It is important for folate, carbohydrate, fat and some protein metabolism and helps maintain a healthy nervous system. Vitamin B12 is essential for synthesis of the genetic material, DNA.

Vitamin C – A vitamin that is essential for the formation of connective tissue, bones and teeth. It is important for wound healing and gum tissue health and assists in fat breakdown (fat metabolism). Vitamin C enhances iron absorption and provides antioxidant properties.

Vitamin D – An essential vitamin that promotes normal bone and tooth formation. It stimulates calcium and phosphorous absorption and is essential for their metabolism. Scientists believe that vitamin D has other functions unrelated to calcium. A variety of cells not involved with calcium metabolism, including certain immune cells, utilize vitamin D for purposes that are not yet understood.

Vitamin E – An essential vitamin that works as an antioxidant to protect cells, vitamin A and unsaturated fatty acids. It also plays a role in maintaining healthy red blood cells.

Vitamin K – An essential vitamin that helps synthesize proteins involved in normal blood clotting. It is also needed for the synthesis of a key protein in bone formation and may play a role in reducing hip fractures.

Water – An essential nutrient for life. It helps eliminate toxic materials in the body, transports nutrients in the body and body fluids and dissipates excess heat through perspiration.

Zinc – A trace mineral that is essential for proper growth and development and is involved in protein synthesis and digestion, wound healing, bone health and the synthesis of genetic material, DNA. It also modulates immune function and is a key component in a major antioxidant enzyme in the body.

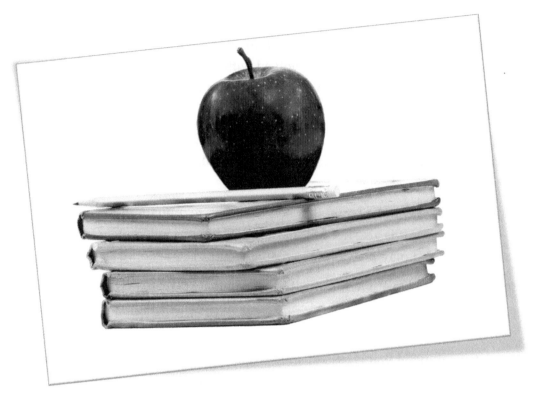

Invest a few moments in thinking.
It will pay good dividends.
— Anonymous

Chapter 17

References

Chapter 2: September – Family Meals

Food and Nutrition Board, Institute of Medicine. *Food Marketing to Children and Youth: Threat or Opportunity?* Washington, DC: The National Academies Press; 2005. Available at: http://books.nap.edu.

Fulkerson JA, Story M, Mellin A, et al. Family dinner meal frequency and adolescent development: relationships with developmental assets and high-risk behaviors. *J Adolesc Health*. 2006;39:337-345.

Fulkerson JA, Story M, Neumark-Sztainer D, Rydell S. Family meals: perceptions of benefits and challenges among parents of 8- to 10-year-old children. *J Am Diet Assoc.* 2008;108:706-709.

Stanford Prevention Research Center, Stanford University School of Medicine. Building "generation play": addressing the crisis of inactivity among America's children. 2007. Available at: http://hip.stanford.edu/documents.

Chapter 3: October – Feeding the Growing Brain

Agricultural Research Service, United States Department of Agriculture. National Nutrient Database for Standard Reference, Release 24. Available at: http://www.ars.usda.gov.

Campolongo P, Roozendaal B, Trezza, et al. Fat-induced satiety factor oleoylethanolamide enhances memory consolidation. *Proc Natl Acad Sci.* 2009;106:8027-8031.

Food and Nutrition Board, Institute of Medicine. *Dietary Reference Intakes for Thiamin, Riboflavin, Niacin, Vitamin B6, Folate, Vitamin B12, Pantothenic Acid, Biotin and Choline.* Washington, DC: National Academy Press; 1998.

Kris-Etherton PM, Taylor DS, Yu-Poth S, et al. Polyunsaturated fatty acids in the food chain in the United States. *Am J Clin Nutr.* 2000;71(suppl 1):179-188.

Rampersaud GC, Pereira MA, Girard BL, et al. Breakfast habits, nutritional status, body weight, and academic performance in children and adolescents. *JAMA.* 2005:105:743-760.

Riediger ND, Othman RA, Suh M, Moghadasian MH. A systemic review of the roles of n-3 fatty acids in health and disease. *J Am Diet Assoc.* 2009;109:668-679.

Sears B. *The Omega Rx Zone: The Miracle of High-Dose Fish Oil.* New York, NY: HarperCollins Publisher, Inc.; 2002.

Chapter 4: November – Eat Your Colors

Agricultural Research Service, United States Department of Agriculture. National Nutrient Database for Standard Reference, Release 24. Lycopene Nutrient List. Available at: http://www.ars.usda.gov.

Bagchi D, Sen CK, Bagchi M, Atalay M. Anti-angiogenic, antioxidant, and anti-carcinogenic properties of a novel anthocyanin-rich berry extract formula. *Biochemistry.* 2004;69:75-80.

Center for Disease Control and Prevention. Third national health and nutrition examination survey (NHANES III), 1988-1994. Available at: http://www.cdc.gov/nchs/nhanes.htm.

Center for Nutrition Policy and Promotion, United States Department of Agriculture. ChooseMyPlate National Nutrition Education Campaign. Available at: http://www.choosemyplate.gov.

Dole Food Company. *Encyclopedia of Foods: A Guide to Healthy Nutrition.* San Diego, Calif: Elsevier Science and Technology Books; 2002.

Environmental Working Group. Shoppers guide to pesticides. Available at: http://www.foodnews.org.

Fruits and Vegetables More Matters. What fruits & vegetables are in season? Available at: http://www.fruitsandveggiesmorematters.org.

Greer B. A guide to buying fresh fruits and vegetables. Available at: http://www.utextension.utk.edu.

Joseph JA, Shukitt-Hale B, Denisova NA, et al. Reversals of age-related declines in neuronal signal transduction, cognitive, and motor behavioral deficits with blueberry, spinach, or strawberry dietary supplementation. *J Neurosci.* 1999;19:8114-8121.

Lu C, Toepel K, Irish K, et al. Organic diets significantly lower children's dietary exposure to organophosphorus pesticides. *Environ Health Perspect.* 2006;114:260-263.

Magkos F, Arvaniti F, Zampelas A. Organic food: nutritious food or food for thought? A review of the evidence. *Int J Food Sci Nutr.* 2003;54:357-371.

Manach C, Scalbert A, Morand C, et al. Polyphenols: food sources and bioavailability. *Am J Clin Nutr.* 2004;79:727-747.

Spill MK, Birch LL, Roe LS, Rolls BJ. Eating vegetables first: using portion size to increase children's vegetable intake. *Obesity.* 2009;17(suppl 2):S63-S64.

United States Department of Agriculture, University of Minnesota Nutrition Coordinating Center. USDA-NCC Carotenoid Database for US Foods: 1998. Available at: http://www.nalusda.gov/fnic/foodcomp/Data/car98/car98.html.

Wansink B. *Mindless Eating.* New York, NY: Bantam Dell; 2006.

Wu X, Beecher GR, Holden JM, et al. Concentration of anthocyanins in common foods in the United States and estimations of normal consumption. *J Agric Food Chem.* 2006;54:4069-4075.

Chapter 5: December – De-Stress, Sleep and Learn

Huang D, Ou B, Prior RL. The chemistry behind antioxidant capacity assays. *J Agric Food Chem.* 2005;53:1841-1856.

National Sleep Foundation. Children and sleep. Available at: http://www.sleepfoundation.org.

Walker MP, Stickgold R. Sleep-dependent learning and memory consolidation. *Neuron.* 2004;44:121-133.

Chapter 6: January – Pack a Power Lunch

Greenwood CE, Winocur G. High-fat diets, insulin resistance and declining cognitive function. *Neurobiol Aging.* 2005;26(suppl 1):42-45.

Chapter 7: February – Kids in the Kitchen

Bell KI, Tepper BJ. Short-term vegetable intake by young children classified by 6-n-propylthoiuracil bitter-taste phenotype. *Am J Clin Nutr.* 2006;84:245-251.

Cooke LJ, Haworth CM, Wardle J. Genetic and environmental influences on children's food neophobia. *Am J Clin Nutr.* 2007;86:428-433.

Fisher JO, Mennella JA, Hughes SO, Mendoza PM, Patrick H. Offering "dip" promotes intake of a moderately-liked raw vegetable among preschoolers with genetic sensitivity to bitterness. *J Acad Nutr Dietetics.* 2012;112:235-245.

Kaminski LC, Henderson SA, Drewnowski A. Young women's food preferences and taste responsiveness to 6-n-propylthiouracil (PROP). *Physiol Behav.* 2000;68:691-697.

Keller KL, Steinmann L, Nurse RJ, Tepper BJ. Genetic taste sensitivity to 6-n-propylthiouracil influences food preference and reported intake in preschool children. *Appetite.* 2002;38:3-12.

Chapter 8: March – Fit Body, Fit Brain

Academy of Nutrition and Dietetics. Sports nutrition: tips for fueling athletes. 2006. Available at: http://www.eatright.org.

Beilock SL, Lyons IM, Mattarella-Micke A, Nusbaum HC, Small SL. Sports experience changes the neural processing of action language. *Proc Natl Acad Sci.* 2008;105:13269-13273.

Clarke DD, Sokoloff L. Circulation and energy metabolism of the brain. In: Siegel GJ, Agranoff BW, Albers RW, Fischer SK, Uhler MD, eds. *Basic Neurochemistry: Molecular, Cellular and Medical Aspects.* 6th ed. Philadelphia, Pa: Lippincott-Raven; 1999.

Davis CL, Tomporowski PD, Boyle CA, et al. Effects of aerobic exercise on overweight children's cognitive functioning: a randomized controlled trial. *Res Q Exerc Sport.* 2007;78:510–519.

Department of Health and Human Services, United States Department of Agriculture. Dietary Guidelines for Americans, 2010. Available at: http://www.health.gov/dietaryguidelines/2010.asp.

Fisher JO. Effects of age on children's intake of large and self-selected food portions. *Obesity.* 2007;15:403-412.

Geier AB, Foster GD, Womble LG, et al. The relationship between relative weight and school attendance among elementary schoolchildren. *Obesity.* 2007;15:2157-2161.

Orlet Fisher J, Rolls BJ, Birch LL. Children's bite size and intake of an entree are greater with large portions than with age-appropriate or self-selected portions. *Am J Clin Nutr*. 2003;77:1164-1170.

Roberts CK, Freed B, McCarthy W. Low aerobic fitness and obesity are associated with lower standardized test scores in children. *J Pediatr*. 2010;156:711-718.

Stanford Prevention Research Center, Stanford University School of Medicine. Building "generation play": addressing the crisis of inactivity among America's children. 2007. Available at: http://hip.stanford.edu/documents.

Tudor-Locke C, Pangrazi RP, Corbin CB, et al. BMI-referenced standards for recommended pedometer-determined steps/day in children. *Prev Med*. 2004;38:857-864.

Chapter 9: April – Celebration Beyond Cupcakes

Academy of Nutrition and Dietetics. Position of the American Dietetic Association: use of nutritive and nonnutritive sweeteners. *J Am Diet Assoc*. 2004;104(2):255-275.

Burt B. The use of sorbitol- and xylitol-sweetened chewing gum in caries control. *J Am Dent Assoc*. 2006;137:190-196.

Johnson RK, Appel LJ, Brands M, et al, for the American Heart Association Nutrition Committee of the Council on Nutrition, Physical Activity, and Metabolism and the Council on Epidemiology and Prevention. Dietary sugars intake and cardiovascular health: a scientific statement from the American Heart Association. *Circulation*. 2009;120(11):1011-1020.

Molteni R, Barnard RJ, Ying Z, Roberts CK, Gómez-Pinilla F. A high-fat, refined sugar diet reduces hippocampal brain-derived neurotrophic factor, neuronal plasticity, and learning. *Neuroscience*. 2002;112:803-814.

Pennington JAT. *Bowes & Church's Food Values of Portions Commonly Used*. 17th ed. JB Lippincott Company: Philadelphia, Pa; 1998.

Chapter 10: May – New Foods for Curious Minds

Cooke LJ, Haworth CM, Wardle J. Genetic and environmental influences on children's food neophobia. *Am J Clin Nutr*. 2007;86:428-433.

Chapter 11: June – The Wonders of Water

Dubois L, Farmer A, Girard M, Peterson K. Regular sugar-sweetened beverage consumption between meals increases risk of overweight among preschool-aged children. *J Am Diet Assoc*. 2007;107:924-935.

FDA Consumer Magazine. Bottle water: better than the tap? July-August 2002. Available at: http://www.fda.gov.

Food and Nutrition Board, Institute of Medicine, National Academies of Health resources pages. Available at: http://www.iom.edu.

Health Canada. Caffeine in Food. Available at: http://www.hc-sc.gc.ca/fn-an/securit/addit/caf/index-eng.php.

Pennington JAT, ed. *Bowes & Church's Food Values of Portions Commonly Used*. 17th ed. JB Lippincott Company: Philadelphia, Pa; 1998.

Sebastian R, Cleveland L, Goldman J, Moshfegh A. Trends in the food intakes of children 1977-2002. *Consumer Interests Annu*. 2006;52: 433-434.

Chapter 12: July – Label Reading Short Cuts

American Heart Association. Know your fats. Available at: http://www.heart.org.

American Heart Association Nutrition Committee, Lichtenstein AH, Appel LJ, Brands M, et al. Diet and lifestyle recommendations revision 2006: a scientific statement from the American Heart Association Nutrition Committee. *Circulation*. 2006;114:82-96.

Anzman SL, Birch LL. Low inhibitory control and restrictive feeding practices predict weight outcomes. *J Pediatr*. 2009;155:651-656.

Department of Health and Human Services, United States Department of Agriculture. Dietary Guidelines for Americans, 2010. Available at: http://www.health.gov/dietaryguidelines/2010.asp.

Fisher JO, Birch LL. Parents' restrictive feeding practices are associated with young girls' negative self-evaluation of eating. *J Am Diet Assoc.* 2000;100:1341-136.

Fisher JO, Birch LL. Restricting access to palatable foods affects children's behavioral response, food selection, and intake. *Am J Clin Nutr.* 1999;69:1264-1272.

Food and Drug Administration. Food labeling; trans fatty acids in nutrition labeling; consumer research to consider nutrient content and health claims and possible footnote or disclosure statements; final rule and proposed rule. *Fed Reg.* 2003;68:41433. Available at: http://www.fda.gov.

Food Marketing Institute. Supermarket facts: industry overview 2008. Available at: http://www.fmi.org/facts_figs/?fuseaction=superfact.

He FJ, Marrero NM, Macgregor GA. Salt and blood pressure in children and adolescents. *J Hum Hypertens.* 2008;22:4-11.

National Academy of Sciences, Institute of Medicine, Food and Nutrition Board. *Dietary Reference Intakes for Water, Potassium, Sodium, Chloride, and Sulfate.* Washington, DC: The National Academies Press; 2004.

United States Department of Agriculture. Empty calories. Available at: http://www.choosemyplate.gov/foodgroups/emptycalories.html.

Zappalla FR, Gidding SS. Lipid management in children. *Endocrinol Metab Clin North Am.* 2009;38:171-183.

Chapter 13: August – Prep for a New School Year

Advance for Occupational Therapy Practitioners. AOTA's national school backpack awareness day is September 22. Available at: http://occupational-therapy.advanceweb.com/Article/AOTAs-National-School-Backpack-Awareness-Day-Is-September-22.aspx.

American Academy of Pediatrics. Back to school tips. Available at: http://www.aap.org/advocacy/releases/augschool.cfm.

American Physical Therapy Association. Backpack safety. Available at: http://www.moveforwardpt.com.

Meals Matter. Healthy back-to-school lunch ideas. Available at: http://www.mealsmatter.org/articles-and-resources/meal-planning-articles/healthy-back-to-school-lunch-ideas.aspx.

Wiersema BM, Wall EJ, Foad SL. Acute backpack injuries in children. *Pediatrics.* 2003;111:163-166.

Chapter 15: Tables, Tips & More

Center for Nutrition Policy and Promotion, United States Department of Agriculture. ChooseMyPlate National Nutrition Education Campaign. Available at: http://www.choosemyplate.gov.

Dudai Y. The neurobiology of consolidations, or, how stable is the engram? *Annu Rev Psychol.* 2004;55:51-86.

Institute of Medicine. *DRI Reference Intakes: The Essential Guide to Nutrient Requirements.* Washington, DC: The National Academies Press; 2006. Available at: http://www.nap.edu/catalog/11537.html.

The NPD Group. National eating trends data. Available at: http://www.npd.com.

Glossary

Campolongo P, Roozendaal B, Trezza V, et al. Fat-induced satiety factor oleoylethanolamide enhances memory consolidation. *Proc Natl Acad Sci U S A.* 2009;106(19):8027-8031.

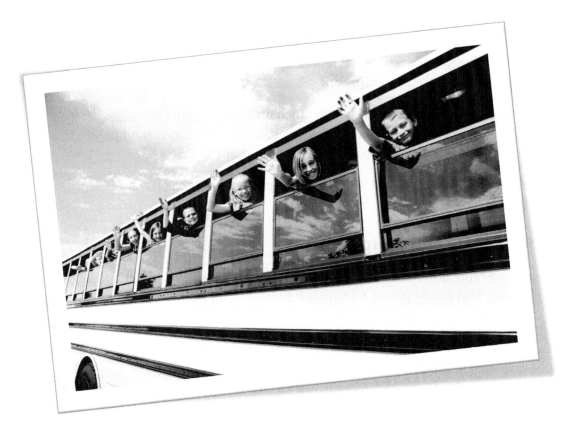

The journey is the reward.
— Chinese proverb

Index

Acknowledgements

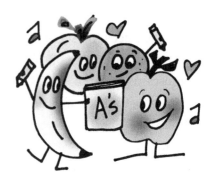

Many thanks to our fearless copy reviewers, Brad Williams, Patti Crandall, Maureen Dunn and Ernest Noble, who provided insightful comments on drafts too numerous to count. Thank you from the bottom of our hearts. You rock!

About the Authors

Kathleen Dunn, MPH, RD, and Lorna Williams, MPH, RD, are registered dietitians who have been collaborating on health and nutrition projects for over 25 years since their graduate school days (Go Bruins!). Lorna's a big fan of a "Make it Fun" approach, while Kathleen gravitates to a "Need to Know" method. It's the perfect blend of whimsy and science to deliver nutrition information that matters to you.

Kathleen and Lorna are members of the Academy of Nutrition and Dietetics (formerly the American Dietetic Association). Kathleen holds a bachelor's degree in biological sciences from the University of California, Irvine, and a master's degree in public health nutrition from the University of California, Los Angeles. Lorna holds two bachelor degrees from the University of California, Berkeley, one in physiology and another in nutrition and food sciences, and a master's degree in public health nutrition from the University of California, Los Angeles.

CPSIA information can be obtained at www.ICGtesting.com
Printed in the USA
LVOW011754031012

301362LV00008B/8/P